The Journey of Perfection

The Journey of Perfection

A Scientific Commentary on
Yoga Sūtras

Original Text Composed by
Sage Pātāñjali

Ashish Dalela

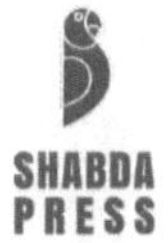

SHABDA
PRESS

The Journey of Perfection—A Scientific Commentary on
Yoga Sūtras
by Ashish Dalela
www.shabda.co

Published by Shabda Press

press.shabda.co
ISBN 978-93-85384-37-0
v1.2 08/2021

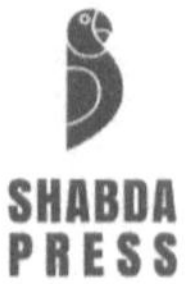

SHABDA
PRESS

CONTENTS

Series Preface

At present, the Vedic philosophical system suffers from many misconceptions—(a) the Vedic texts comprise many disparate or conflicting doctrines that don't form a coherent system, (b) these texts advocate the worship of different deities so the Vedic system must be polytheistic, (c) due to the differences between the various Vedic texts, they must have been authored by different people so they cannot be of divine origin, and (d) the texts produced by various human minds must have originated at different ages and times in history.

Those who want to correct these misconceptions are also making many mistakes. First, they defend the history as being a few thousand years older than modern estimates (when the Vedic tradition is sanātana or eternal). Second, they accept impersonalism as a solution to the supposed polytheism of the Vedas (even though it is solemnly rejected by the Vedic texts). Third, they apologize for the diversity of texts as the intellectual virtue of plural viewpoints (when plurality is different perspectives on a single understanding of reality). Fourth, they visualize Vedic knowledge through the mundane lens of geographical contiguity and genetic resemblances confusing the correction of mistakes with pedestrian ideals of nationalism, political unity, cultural pride, etc., and the true spiritual foundations under which all material identities of body, gender, society, and nation are rejected as a waste of time, are ignored.

This series of books differs from the above-mentioned goals and aspirations. This may potentially reduce the reader list to a smaller number of people who are truly interested in the truth, not a race, nationality, language, etc. But that risk must be taken in the interest of truth, and broader objectives of Vedic knowledge. The sacrifice of immediate interests is hence a necessary evil.

The primary goal of this series of books is to establish that the Vedas constitute a coherent description of reality, which has to be understood from multiple perspectives to grasp its true nature. This understanding can be broadly classified into the following categories—(a) the study of matter as concepts and qualities, (b) the understanding of the soul and its relation to God, (c) the practices by which this nature of the soul and God are practically realized and experienced, and (d) the system of reasoning and logic that is used to explain it to anyone who might be interested. The study of the nature of the soul and God is theology. The practice by which this nature is realized is religion. The description of matter as categories and qualities is philosophy. And the system of reasoning and logic used to explain it to those who are interested is science.

Each perspective can be, in principle, described and understood without the others. For example, we can practice religious mysticism without perfectly knowing theology. We can know the philosophy of reality without religion or theology. And we can understand the science without practicing mysticism.

Nevertheless, the Vedic texts do not put these into separate boxes. Every text discusses all the subjects—science, philosophy, religion, and theology—but with different relative emphases. Some texts are more focused on science, others more on theology and religion, while others more on philosophy. This unifying tendency in the Vedic system is the antithesis of the modern tendency to compartmentalize, separate one issue from another, focus on narrow problems, and create the illusion of progress by going round and round in circles.

The Vedic system looks at all inquiries holistically and their answers to one question cannot contradict the answers to any other potential question. If you progress in philosophy, then you also progress in religion, theology, and science. Scientific progress is not contrary to ethics and morality; spiritual development is not contrary to the necessities of life. The Vedic system is not divided into physics, chemistry, mathematics, sociology, economics, psychology, cosmology, theology, and so on, as its purpose is to create wise people—who know everything—rather than professional academics whose solutions are conceived within the narrow ambits of their primary expertise, rather than broadly concerned with several aspects of the problem needed for a wise person.

The understanding of the knowledge and its application to various areas of human knowledge should be the primary goal because by achieving that goal, the other goals can be achieved automatically. If the knowledge is useful and true, then each path meant to attain it can be useful for people with different abilities and interests. If the Vedic texts describe reality correctly, then the timelessness of the knowledge would be more important than the age of the text. If the philosophy is consistent and complete, then even plural authorship of the texts would indicate a multitude of mutually coherent viewpoints. If the personalistic and aspected nature of reality is understood correctly, then the myriad personalities would not be contradictory to a single person of God. And the universal applicability and the non-sectarian nature of knowledge would make any national, social, cultural, and political pride completely redundant.

Even as the Vedas are divine knowledge, and many times described as the word of God and transmitted through the creator of the universe—Brahma—nobody has to accept their divinity a priori. Vedas recommend faith in the teachers because no student approaches a teacher without some faith. But blind faith—as the antithesis of reason and experience—is rejected. The philosophy of the Vedas is meant to be studied, debated, and discussed by all qualified people (the restriction of the Vedas to a certain class is the restriction of qualification). And the knowledge of the Vedas is beyond race, nation, and society. In all these ways, the Vedas constitute a "secular science"—not atheistic, but secular—as they are amenable to reason and experience, open to sincere inquiry and discussion, and not to be conflated with narrow political objectives.

The primary aim of this series of books is to help the readers understand the knowledge. If the truth of the Vedic texts is known, then we can talk about their history. If the unity of Vedic philosophy is known, then we can talk about whether they had different authors. If by learning this philosophy, we can master every subject, then we can talk about its divine and eternal nature. And if all these are achieved, then we can speak of the intellectual, cultural, and social superiority of the people who have preserved, advanced, and propagated this knowledge selflessly. In fact, by establishing the truth, all other questions about history, authorship, and divinity will become moot—we will accept them without an argument, based on their superiority. Without proving the consistency, completeness, pervasive usefulness, and the empirical truth of this knowledge, there is no point in talking about history, authorship, divinity, geographical heritage, and socio-cultural identities. Without understanding the nature of reality, pride in ancient history makes no difference to the present. And without putting that knowledge into practice, all claims remain the subject of endless subjective opinions and pointless debates. If instead, we focus on the truth in the Vedas, then even the temporaneous goals can also be achieved naturally.

The Vedas in fact describe the history of their appearance, but because people don't believe in the Vedic truth, therefore, they don't accept the history. Because the academics have become accustomed to numerous mythological texts in the West, which were repeatedly modified and curated by religious institutions to suit their political objectives, they think that the Vedas too must be myths. But where is the evidence for the doctoring of the Vedas? We can find that evidence in the case of the Bible and the Koran for instance, where books have been revised many times, and the ideas of the doctors were inserted into the books. But the Vedic tradition gives us no such evidence. Instead, there is clear evidence of the separation of the texts from the commentaries on the texts. The texts are always separate from the commentaries by various authors. Therefore, if we rely on the Vedic texts, we can also understand their own history.

To understand the Six Systems of Philosophy, we need to take note of their historical appearance. The Vedas state that their knowledge has existed since time immemorial, and originated in the four Vedas compiled by Brahma—the creator of the universe—after being inspired in the heart by Lord Viṣṇu. Brahma imparted this knowledge to his sons—the seven sages, Manu, the four Kumaras, and others. These disciples and their successors then produced a broader oral tradition, which was called the "Vedic system"—because it was based on the original four Vedas that were narrated by Brahma to others. This oral tradition was significantly larger than what we know as the Vedic texts today.

Vedic cosmology divides time into cycles of yugas, which are further divided into four sub-ages called Satya-yuga, Treta-yuga, Dvapara-yuga, and Kali-yuga. The Kali-yuga is the smallest age and is 432,000 years. Dvapara is twice that of Kali-yuga, Treta is three times of Kali-yuga, and Satya is four times Kali-yuga. The present age is Kali-yuga. In the bygone ages—Satya, Treta, and Dvapara—which amounts to 3,888,000 solar years, the Vedas existed as an oral tradition, because the people following the system had a great memory.

At the beginning of Kali-yuga, these texts were scribed by Vyāsa, who is also sometimes called Bādarāyana. This is when the oral tradition became a written one. Vyāsa performed a selection from the oral tradition, and the texts he produced by scribing the oral tradition were a subset of the oral tradition.

Vyāsa also divided the oral tradition into many parts, which are today known as Saṃhita, Upaniśad, Tantra, Purāna, Itihāsa, etc. Each of these classes is further divided into many sub-classes and texts. For instance, there are 108 Upaniśad and 18 Purāna. He then also *composed* the Vedānta Sūtra after *compiling* the other Vedic texts. There is a subtle difference between compiling and composing. A compilation is the selective scribing of the oral tradition. But the composition is solely attributable to Bādarāyana (although he often quotes other sages even in this text). Quite simply, Vedānta Sūtra is Bādarāyana's summary of the oral tradition, after the selective scribing of the oral tradition.

While dividing, scribing, and compiling the Vedic texts, Vyāsa referred to the philosophies of some of the Six Systems such as Sāñkhya and Yoga and included them into the Vedic texts. He left out some of the philosophies such as Nyāya, Vaiśeṣika, and Mīmāṃsā as they were, and still are, considered supplementary. We might wonder why. And the answer is that Nyāya is a system of logic, Mīmāṃsā is the use of reason for semantic analysis, and Vaiśeṣika is the application of semantic analysis to the study of material nature. These are, strictly speaking, the applications of Vedic philosophy, which are of great interest to the experts, but not of primary interest to the general population. This exclusion of some philosophies from the primary Vedic texts means that logic, semantic analysis, and its applications to the study of nature, were considered to be not of interest to the people primarily interested in the conclusions.

The selective inclusions and exclusions of some philosophies do not mean that they weren't part of the Vedic tradition. For example, practically everyone undergoing scientific education at present uses logic and mathematics, but the foundations of logic and mathematics are studied only by experts. Similarly, practically everyone masters some language, but the foundations of linguistics are outside the scope for everyone except the experts. The doctors who treat patients learn medicine, but they don't study biochemistry because that is too much unnecessary detail that is not of primary interest to their needs.

Therefore, the inclusion of philosophies of Sāñkhya and Yoga should be viewed as based on the fact that these were considered general information for everyone's use, while the exclusion of philosophies like Nyāya, Vaiśeṣika, and Mīmāṃsā should be viewed as something that was needed only for experts.

Quite separately, complete systems of philosophy existed as the Sūtra texts that this series is about. They were authored by other sages (Sāṅkhya by Kapila, Yoga by Pātañjali, Nyāya by Gautama, Vaiśeṣika by Kanāda, and Mīmāṃsā by Jaimini). These other systems of philosophy are also based on the oral Vedic tradition, which preceded Bādarāyana's selected scribing of the tradition, although Nyāya, Vaiśeṣika, and Mīmāṃsā were not included in the scribing. They too existed as an oral tradition and were scribed by their tradition followers, but their names are not known at present because (a) the texts are relatively small compared to the texts that Vyāsa scribed, and (b) there was no selection performed in the scribing of these texts; they were presented as they were. In that light, we can view Vyāsa as an editor of the Vedic tradition, while the other systems of philosophy had scribes that did not try to edit the Sūtra texts.

The result of this difference between Bādarāyana's selected scribing, and the texts of the other five systems, is that we can sometimes find it hard to cite the claims in the philosophies of Sāṅkhya, Yoga, Nyāya, Vaiśeṣika, and Mīmāṃsā from the Saṃhita, Upaniṣad, Tantra, Purāna, and Itihāsa. This inability to find direct references for one system in another one should not be taken to mean that they are at variance, or that they are not Vedic, or that they were created after the scribing of Vedic texts by other philosophers who did not agree with Bādarāyana's view. We must rather understand that all the Six Systems are based on the oral tradition. Specifically, Sāṅkhya, Yoga, Vaiśeṣika, Nyāya, and Mīmāṃsā had their oral tradition before Bādarāyana scribing a select portion of the oral tradition, followed by composing the Vedānta Sūtra. As far as the historical dates of composing are concerned, Vedānta Sūtra is later. It is for this reason that it is sometimes called Uttara Mīmāṃsā (later analysis).

When we study the Six Systems of philosophy, in one sense, we are studying the much older oral tradition—as it was understood by six different sages. And when we study the Saṃhita, Upaniśad, Tantra, Purāna, and Itihāsa, we are studying the Vedic system as it was selectively scribed by Bādarāyana. The differences in these systems do not indicate a contradiction, but the fact that the oral tradition was bigger than the combinations of all the texts at present.

The point is this: The Six Systems are Vedic because they are all based on the oral tradition. They are also Vedic because Bādarāyana's texts directly reference Sāṅkhya and Yoga, which are also referenced by Nyāya, Vaiśeṣika, and Mīmāṃsā. Then, several doctrines about the nature of the soul and God are common across the Six Systems and can be found in Bādarāyana's texts. Therefore, the Six Systems are not divergent philosophies, but different streams within the oral tradition that emphasized different aspects, and were thereby encoded as the Sūtra texts, that came to be studied by different students, and that inherited method of teacher-disciple succession created many schools.

And yet, there is widespread perception at present that the Six Systems of Philosophy are divergent, or even contradictory. This perception of divergence is not entirely fictional; it is indeed based on fact. But its appearance is relatively recent. Such deviations appear in the age of Kaliyuga, where people tend to replace understanding with argument, and incommensurate ideas that deviate from the Vedic philosophy appear. To support their contentions, they also reject many essential aspects of the cohesive system of philosophy.

To understand this divergence, we need to consider the last few thousand years of history, in which three philosophies—materialism, voidism, and impersonalism—have dominated. Each of the Six Systems of Philosophy rejects these doctrines. The world, in Vedic philosophy, reflects the properties of God like a mirror reflects a person's image. The mirror is real, and hence, matter is real. The form in the mirror is objective—the image in the mirror is real. Similarly, the reflection in the mirror is not a creation of the mirror, or an illusion, because there is a person outside the mirror. Since there is a transcendent person, therefore, the mirror and the reflection in it are not the only reality; there is also a transcendent reality. By acknowledging a transcendent reality, materialism is rejected. By acknowledging that this transcendent reality is a person, impersonalism is rejected. And by recognizing that the person exists even if not reflected in the mirror—i.e., if the world doesn't exist—voidism is rejected.

The Six Systems texts delve into the details of why materialism, voidism, and impersonalism are false. They describe why God desires to see His reflection—namely, that it is a process of self-awareness and self-cognition. They describe how God is reflected in the mirror—the mirror is also a person, not an impersonal thing; the reflection in the mirror is the mirror "knowing" God; the mirror is then identified as God's energy or Śakti, and two realities—one masculine and the other feminine—are seen as the basis of the world. The immense variety in the reflection is attributed to the myriad aspects of God, which are integrated in God but separated in the Śakti. Thus, the created world is called *duality* whereas God is described as *non-duality*. The separation of the integrated reality is then understood as a mechanism by which God knows Himself—quite like a person looking into a mirror to see his varied features.

Each of the Six Systems of Vedic philosophy goes over these themes in different orders, emphasizing different aspects of this ideology, dwelling more on some things and less on others. Each philosophy refutes impersonalism, voidism, and materialism as these doctrines are contrary to the Vedic system.

In the modern context, the criticism of materialism can be equated to the rejection of modern science, and the ideas that underpin it. The Six Systems texts provide alternative descriptions of matter too, unparalleled by any other system in the past or present in its breadth and cohesiveness. The methods of realizing the truth of this description—i.e., the methods for practical and empirical confirmations—are also presented. The alternative to materialism is hence also rational and empirical, and without changing the definition of science—i.e., empirical, and rational truth—the reality is presented differently. It is rather the change of the doctrine of matter, with far wider empiricism, that covers the experiences of the senses, mind, intellect, ego, and the moral sense. The criticism of materialism therefore also constitutes an alternative science.

Similarly, in the modern context, the criticism of voidism can be equated to the rejection of Buddhism and allied traditions, which reject the reality of the soul and God. This rejection, similar to the rejection of materialism, is relatively easier, and the Six Systems of Philosophy don't dwell upon it as much.

The greatest focus in these systems—apart from the description of their position on the nature of reality—is to distinguish it from impersonalism because impersonalism uses more Vedic terminology than voidism. All over the Six Systems texts, we can find the rejection of all the contentions of impersonalism, namely—(a) that nature is a deluding agency, (b) that nature is inert, (c) that Oneness is the ultimate reality instead of diversity, (d) that this Oneness is formless, (e) that the desire and individuality of the soul are temporary.

All the followers of the Vedic tradition easily accept the rejections of materialism and voidism, but the rejection of impersonalism has become contentious because impersonalism used to be a non-Vedic system until

Shankaracharya authored a commentary on the Vedānta Sūtra, to establish that impersonalism was Vedic. This commentary replaced the void of the Buddhists with two realities—called Brahman and māyā—with Brahman being an undivided consciousness, and māyā being inert matter (sort of like the Cartesian mind-body dualism). Since Brahman is undivided, therefore, the analogy of a person reflected in a mirror is modified to say that the mirror—i.e., māyā—creates an illusory picture of the formless. Since māyā is originally formless, and Brahman is always formless, this doctrine runs into difficulties in explaining the origin of forms. Calling something an illusion doesn't make it go away. The doctrine might also sometimes say that even māyā is a conscious entity, which deliberately tries to mislead Brahman into an illusion. This is also problematic, because if māyā is a deluding agency, then everything in the world—including the Vedic scriptures—must be illusory, as they are byproducts of māyā. The evil nature of māyā would entail that Brahman can never be liberated out of māyā because even the supposed sources of enlightenment are merely delusions.

The fact is that Vedānta does not support such an interpretation, because there are explicit statements about devotion to the Lord, the difference between the soul and God, and the divine relationship between God and His Sakti. Hence, Shankaracharya's commentary was an ill-conceived misrepresentation. His position was, in fact, subsequently criticized by other Vedānta views, and owing to these successive interpretations, the Vedānta system is popular today.

The Vedic practitioners of that time could have protested Shankaracharya's commentary, but they welcomed it on pragmatic grounds—they saw Indian society afflicted by Buddhism and considered that to be a bigger and more urgent problem. In voidism, every book is a delusion, because the whole world is unreal. Therefore, even the Vedas must be a delusion. Shankaracharya argued against that idea, and his key contribution was to explain why the Vedic texts are not delusions. But he married an un-Vedic doctrine of impersonalism to the acceptance of the Vedic texts as divine knowledge and divine authority.

To support his impersonal doctrine, Shankaracharya also created a schism between the Six Systems, rejecting the other five systems in his Vedānta commentary. Shankaracharya could not comment on Vedānta alone, if the integrity of the other five systems of philosophy—namely, Sāñkhya, Mīmāṃsā, Nyāya, Vaiśeṣika, and Yoga—wasn't challenged.

Historically, these six systems had always supported each other and used each other's doctrines. The schism between the Six Systems of philosophy owes to the criticism of the other five systems by Shankaracharya. Since that time, people began to consider the Six Systems as divergent and inconsistent philosophies, and their teachers began to grow apart, instead of being considered a part of a single coherent system.

Even as later Ācharyas tried to correct this problem by commenting again on Vedānta Sūtra, the results were less than desirable. Three specific problems arose quickly out of these successive commentaries. First, the commentaries of Rāmanujāchārya, Mādhavāchārya, and others, emphasized the worship of Lord Viṣṇu, instead of Lord Śiva, thus creating a schism between Vaishnavism and Shaivism. Second, they restricted themselves to the discussion of the soul and God, neglecting His Śakti. Third, the study of material nature and Śakti was embraced by the Tantra system, and the Vedic system split again into the third sect of Shaktism, which seemed different from Shaivism and Vaishnavism.

The specific outcome of Shankaracharya's commentary was the schism between the Six Systems, and the specific outcome of the later commentaries was the schism between Vaishnavism, Shaivism, and Shaktism. Once these two types of schisms were created, the unity in the Vedic system was effectively lost. The Vaishnavas and Shaivas focused on Vedānta, and the Shaktas took a greater interest in the other five systems of philosophy. Over time, each of these three systems was further split into many subsects, each based on different Vedic texts, but each of them neglecting the principles presented in the other texts. To the outsider, this reinforced the belief that the Vedic system is not just diverse but also disparate; that it is a collection of many contradictory ideologies.

These schisms continue to play havoc on the understanding of the Vedic system even today. For instance, Sāñkhya is included in all Puranas, but practically everyone who reads these Puranas glosses over Sāñkhya and proceeds into the stories because the teachers of the Puranas are mostly Vaishnavas and they deemphasize everything other than select aspects of Vedānta. Similarly, the discussion of Yoga forms a core aspect of all the Upanishads, but the teachers of these Upanishads, who are mostly Shaivas, gloss over Yoga philosophy because they are focused on Vedānta. When outsiders look at these discrepancies, they find it justifiable to create even more discrepancies. For instance, the Yoga Sūtra doesn't speak about the Kundalini, although Tantra does. There is no discussion about

Chakras in the Yoga Sūtra, although it is present in the Tantras. The Yoga Sūtra speaks of only one Asana or meditative posture, while Tantras speak of 8,400,000 such postures. While Tantra practitioners indulge in sexual practices, the Yoga Sūtra speaks of celibacy. While Yoga Sūtra rejects the pursuit of mystical powers, the Tantra system advocates it. The modern practitioners of Yoga have therefore effectively transformed it into Tantra. This means that even more people who are interested in the transcendental nature of the Six Systems of Philosophy, are repelled from it, as it is now Tantric.

The schisms between the various systems are also exacerbated because the Vedānta school emphasizes the urgency of liberation from the material world, while other systems discuss the nature of the material world. If you think of the material world as a raging firestorm, then Vedānta says that you must quickly get out of it. Sāñkhya explains how the fire started. Yoga explains how to get out of the firestorm. Nyāya explains how that fire is a logical outcome of the incompatibility between soul and matter. Vaiśeṣika explains how the fire burns. And Mīmāṃsā discusses the protections while trying to get out of the firestorm. Now, it is up to the reader to decide— Do you want to treat the methods of protecting yourself against the fire as a recommendation for permanently living in the fire, or a method to defend yourself while you are trying to escape? Do you want to consider the description of fire and how it burns just an intellectual curiosity or urgent information that matches the urge to escape the fire?

The divergences in the Six Systems are exacerbated when their position in the larger scheme of things is not understood. Then, a method for protection against the burning fire is treated as a recommendation to stay in the fire. Or, information about the fire's burning is used just for intellectual curiosity. This recommendation then is seen as a contrast against the exhortation to escape the fire, and, lo and behold, a contradiction between the texts is produced.

To avoid such misinterpretations, one must study all the Six Systems, because that gives one the conviction that there is a fire (in case you don't believe it), there is a reason why it was started (in case you are looking for a rational justification), there is a method to escape it, and there are methods to avoid its harmful effects while you are trying to run out of the firestorm. Wearing a mask is not contradictory to running out; understanding that the fire will not die on its own is not contradictory to deciding that one must run out of the fire. In this way, the Six Systems of philosophy are consistent and coherent, despite their diverging emphases. By studying them, we obtain a view into the larger oral tradition, how this tradition was adapted for different purposes, and why all the systems of philosophy are important for different aspects of the problem. These books are the manuals for life—useful for different kinds of issues.

Finally, a few words must be said about the prevalent commentaries, and how the present commentaries differ. The prevalent commentaries today fall into two broad categories. First, experts in one system, trained by their tradition, comment on only one system of philosophy. Second, academics not trained in any system by the tradition, but having some expertise in the Sanskrit language, comment on multiple systems; they produce false interpretations of things that they don't understand because the context in which the text is written completely escapes them. Both these classes seem interesting to historians, but they mean little to most people because their ideas are not compared to modern thinking. The experts are restricted to one system; the non-experts are misleading; and neither experts nor non-experts demonstrate the relevance of an ancient system in a modern world—when so much around has changed.

These commentaries aim to carry out an unthinkable marriage between (a) the text, (b) the broader Vedic context, (c) demonstrate how this knowledge is relevant today, and (d) make it assimilable to people who know little about Vedic philosophy (or even about Western philosophy and modern science).

This series of books is subtitled "Scientific Commentaries", by which I mean reason and experience—something that can be rationally explained, put into practice, and confirmed by experience. I also mean a contrast or similarity to modern science, Western philosophy, and other prevalent systems of thinking. The former is meant to demonstrate that this is not based on "faith"—although enough faith is needed to read the books, put some of it in practice, and realize the truth. The latter is meant to assist the understanding of the modern mind which is accustomed to almost everything other than Vedic doctrines.

We progress from what we know to what we don't. If what we know is true, then it must be confirmed. If what we know is false, then it must be rejected by reason and evidence. The books are meant to provide adequate background to help people understand. This is a different approach to commentaries than those that have been done in the past: The past commentators relied exclusively on referencing other Vedic texts, and that was acceptable in a society where the Vedic texts were popular and their tenets were accepted. It is not useful for a global audience, or those who are educated in modern science but know very little about Vedic texts. They need an alternative, and these books can help.

From an academic viewpoint, the purpose of writing scientific commentaries is also to transform the discussion of Vedic texts from one of history, linguistics, and religious studies to one about science, philosophy, and empirical merit. Unless Vedic texts are seen as technical information, rather than poetry and literature, their content cannot be truly evaluated and appreciated.

Any ambitious project is hard, and anything hard is likely to have flaws. But it is said that thoroughly honest people enjoy and appreciate reading about the truth even if imperfectly composed. I sincerely hope that you will too.

Book Preface

The Yoga system of philosophy dwells on the following key topics:

- The understanding of the nature of chitta, which is an unconscious repository of impressions from the past. We can understand these impressions as the ideas that were acquired in previous lives. The Yoga system describes how successive manifestations from the chitta produce the mind, the senses, and eventually the body. This produced reality then binds the soul, quite like a spider who might produce a web and then seem to be caught in its own creation. Therefore, the Yoga system prescribes the processes by which the successive productions of the modifications of chitta can be stopped. That cessation would then lead to the soul's liberation.

- It discusses the eight-fold path of meditation called aṣtānga-yoga. The eight limbs of this process are called Yama, Niyama, Āsana, Pranāyāma, Pratyāhara, Dhārana, Dhyāna, and Samādhi. The system prescribes only one Āsana, and many types of Yama and Niyama. This is quite instructive to the modern practitioners who don't practice the Yama (don'ts of life) and Niyama (do's of life), but only practice many types of Āsana. The Yoga system also describes the preconditions of meditation, namely, the perfection of Pranāyāma, and the progression from Dhārana, which is an initial impression, to Dhyāna, which is detailed understanding of the object of the meditation, to Samādhi, which is seeing oneself as the part of the object of meditation. The first five steps are said to be external, while the next three steps are said to be internal. The first five steps are also different compared to other processes of spiritual upliftment described in Sāñkhya, and the last three are common.

Thus, the eight-fold path is not different in its goals, although appears to be different in the initial stages of the practice.

- The Yoga philosophy repeatedly emphasizes devotion and surrender to the Lord. This is initially presented as the method of the perfection of yoga, then it is presented as the goal of the perfection of yoga, then it is presented as the practice of those who have previously perfected yoga, and finally it is presented as the state after the perfection of yoga is attained. Based on these statements, the devotion to the Lord is established as a process, a goal, a proven path, and the final conclusion by those who are perfected. The repeated emphasis establishes this as the ultimate view of yoga.

- The text refutes impersonal ideas about the cessation of all qualities upon the perfection of yoga. It describes how the perfection leads to the development of spiritual senses by which the Paramātma is perceived, and these are produced from within the soul. The text discusses numerous spiritual qualities of the soul, and states that these qualities are pure forms of meaning, thereby rejecting the contention that these may be material qualities. The text rejects many popular meditations on emptiness or a void, the cessation of thoughts, or a merger of various consciousnesses. All these are recognized as possible states, but not considered ultimate or even permanent states. Thus, a difference between voidistic, impersonalistic, and truly divine meditations is established.

- There is a discussion about the various material advancements obtained by the yoga process, such as a strong body, freedom from illness, place in heavenly planets, knowledge of the nature of the sun, moon, and the stars, and eight types of mystical perfections. However, two things are noted subsequently. First, by the time these perfections are attained, the desire for enjoyment is almost completely destroyed. Second, the remnants of the desire to enjoy, the text warns, can lead to a fall from the position of perfection. Thus, even though such perfections are noted, they are indirectly discouraged as not being the real purpose of the yoga practice. They are, however, recommended as a method by which bodily strength leads to mental and emotional strength, and the latter then brings about the courage to tolerate the difficulties of yoga. The mystical perfections are thus recommended for a person who lacks mental and emotional strength to tolerate difficulties.

The study of the above key areas in the Yoga Sūtra refutes some of the common misconceptions about its practices today. First, the emphasis on postures is contrary to the system; there is far greater emphasis on renunciation, celibacy, cleanliness, and truthfulness. Second, all the impersonal doctrines about the merger of the soul into the Supreme Soul or Paramātma are summarily rejected. Third, the manifest differences between the aṣṭānga-yoga and other systems are only in the so-called "external" aspects of body control, and not in the "internal" aspects of meditation, where devotion to the Lord is the sole conclusion.

Finally, we might note in passing that there is absolutely no discussion of Chakras, Kundalini, and other bodily aspects of the yoga process, with which people today are preoccupied. These latter practices are based on the Tantra system, rather than on Yoga Sūtra. Those who follow such practices, therefore, are not practicing Yoga philosophy, but a system of Tantric practices. Tantra practices have also become popular among the Buddhists, who borrowed these from the Vedic Tantra system, and merged them into their voidistic philosophy. The Tantra system is considered much lower than the Yoga system. Just as mystic perfections are means to an end in Yoga, similarly, the Tantra practices are a means to an end for those who cannot practice Yama and Niyama. For instance, if someone cannot practice celibacy, then they are prescribed an alternative system of sex by which sexual enjoyment is severely curtailed. If someone cannot practice solitude and silence, then they are given an elaborate ritual by which to engage their mind through an activity performed by the body. The postures and practices used in Tantra are not Yoga, but they have also been practiced by those who found the stipulations of Yoga Sūtra impossible to implement.

CHAPTER 1

Sūtra 1.1
अथ योगानुशासनम्
atha yogānuśāsanam

atha—now; yoga—yoga; anuśāsanam—the instruction.

TRANSLATION

Now, the instructions of the union.

COMMENTARY

The term yoga means 'union'. The question arises: Union with what? As we will see later in the text, it is the union between the soul and the Supreme Soul. The next question arises: If they are to be united, why are they currently separated? The answer is that both the soul and the Supreme Soul have free will. If the free will of the soul acts independently of the free will of the Supreme Soul, then they are called separated, although there is no physical separation. But if the free will of the soul acts in accordance with the will of the Supreme Soul, then they are said to be united, although there is no physical union. Thus, we must distinguish the physical ideas of union and separation from the idea of 'union' here because we are not talking about physical things. We are talking about two persons— the soul and the Supreme Soul—which are eternally distinct. However, the Supreme Soul exists in everything as the purpose of those things—the purpose indicates how that thing must be used, and the intended use of each thing is also called their *dharma* or duty. When our life is lived in accordance with the intended purpose of our existence, then that life is considered yoga and dharma. If our life's purpose is different from the intended purpose, then it is not yoga and dharma. The union with the Supreme Soul is therefore recognizing that we have an intended purpose, which cannot be invented whimsically, as it exists in each thing, and person. When the purpose of our life becomes the intended purpose, that is yoga. It is a merger of the *purpose* of the soul with the Supreme Soul, not a merger of the soul with the Supreme Soul.

Sūtra 1.2
योगश्चित्तवृत्तनिरोधः
yogaścittavṛttinirodhaḥ

yoga—the yoga; citta—the chitta; vṛtti—the modifications; nirodhaḥ—the cessation.

TRANSLATION

By yoga, the cessation of the modifications of the chitta is achieved.

COMMENTARY

The soul's cognitive capacity is called *chit* and its preliminary material representation is the *chitta*. In this preliminary form, the chitta is the combination of two things—(a) the primordial material energy called pradhāna in Sāñkhya, and (b) the individual history of each soul, which his called niyati in Sāñkhya. The pradhāna is the idea of being the lord, master, leader, or boss, and when it is combined with the history, it becomes a unique individual idea of lordship, mastery, leadership, or bossiness. The pradhāna is the collection of all possible notions of mastery, and the chitta is an individual subset of these ideas (based on a person's history). Therefore, the chitta is a subset of the pradhāna.

From the chitta arise the material desires, which are different ways to exhibit the mastery, and they are called prakṛti. The term prakṛti has two variations—cosmic and individual. Cosmic prakṛti is the balanced state of the three modes (sattva, rajas, and tamas) and it is manifest from pradhāna; it denotes a mastery that is also balanced in all the qualities. Then, the individual prakṛti is a product of the cosmic prakṛti, which is not balanced, but an individual idea of mastery. For example, the individual prakṛti constitutes a particular soul's ideas about a specific type of mastery, whereas the cosmic prakṛti is the mastery in everything because the three modes of prakṛti are balanced within it. Thus, it is sometimes said that the pradhāna manifests a prakṛti, and the individual's history or niyati is mixed with that prakṛti to create an individual persona.

The chitta is that personal history-imbued persona, and it is unique to each person. When this chitta gives rise to desires, then these products of chitta are also called prakṛti, but it is the individual's, rather than cosmic prakṛti. The sense of individual mastery takes on many forms. For example, one person may consider knowledge as mastery, while another person might think that wealth is mastery. These ideas about what it means to be a master are called the mahattattva or the essence of greatness. Once these ideals have been chosen, then the ego is manifest, which says: You may be seeking some mastery, but you are already great and deserving of that mastery. This sense of deserved mastery or entitlement is the ego. The ego gives rise to specific goals by which mastery will be demonstrated—to oneself and the others. So, pradhāna is the idea that we are capable of mastery. The prakṛti is a specific idea of mastery. The mahattattva is the idea of greatness—which if possessed—will rationalize the mastery. And the ego is the entitlement for a person to pursue that mastery.

All these together constitute what people call "the pursuit of life and happiness", which is a euphemism for (a) being capable of enjoyment, (b) having a choice for enjoyment, (c) having the great qualities to enjoy, and (d) the entitlement to pursue enjoyment. The entitlement for enjoyment therefore has three preliminary conditions. First, there is a recognition that I am capable of enjoyment, which comes from pradhāna. Second, there is the acceptance that I have a choice to select a type of enjoyment, which comes from prakṛti. And third, that I am deserving of enjoyment, which comes from mahattattva. Within the ego, or the entitlement, therefore, are three things—deserving, desiring, and ability. When the soul enters the material world, and sees pradhāna, it realizes that it can enjoy. Then, he chooses a particular type of enjoyment. And then he tries to get the qualities due to which he would be deserving of enjoyment. Finally, when he has the ability, the desire, and great qualities, then he says: Now that I have acquired the great qualities, and I have chosen to enjoy a certain way, and I am capable of enjoyment, therefore, I am *entitled* to enjoyment.

We can illustrate these by an example of a writer. The writer must initially recognize that he is capable of writing. Then, he must choose a particular type of writing—e.g., fiction or non-fiction, in some specific genre. Then, he must acquire the knowledge and the art of writing. Finally, when he has acquired the knowledge and art, then he says: I am now entitled to write on a subject.

The chitta is the ability to write, and it comes from pradhāna combined with a history. We can call this history the skills or abilities we have acquired in the past. Based on these skills, a desire springs, from that desire, some type of greatness is acquired, and from those great qualities, an entitlement develops. The development of desires, greatness, and entitlement is the gradual manifestation of the chitta, and it is called the modification of the chitta. If a person is convinced that they are incapable of doing something, then they don't get the desire, they don't acquire the great qualities, and they don't develop the entitlement. Therefore, a person must be convinced that something is feasible for them. People who have a good past, and are born in good families, and receive a good nurturing, tend to believe in their ability to create a better future, by acquiring great qualities, and have the entitlement to pursue those goals. Conversely, those who have a bad past think that success is impossible. They don't develop desires, don't try to acquire greatness, and don't have the entitlement. However, at the root of these things lies the absence of self-confidence.

The purpose of yoga is to terminate the successive manifestation of desires, material greatness, and entitlement to enjoy, and the purification of chitta is obtained when the chitta is purified of the idea that I am capable of enjoyment. A person who suffers from impotence doesn't get the desire for sex, he doesn't pursue the greatness that will make him or her attractive to the opposite sex, and doesn't consider himself or herself entitled to receive the attention of the opposite sex. Therefore, when the recognition of ability is destroyed, then all successive manifestations from that ability are also destroyed. This ability is also sometimes called 'power', and the material energy is also called Śakti or the power of the Lord. The Lord delegates this power to the soul, and it becomes an entrapment because the soul thinks that it is meant for him to enjoy.

If the Lord takes away this ability, then desires, greatness, and entitlement are automatically destroyed, because the soul finds itself incapable of this enjoyment. However, the destruction of desires due to impotence is not the permanent solution. The permanent solution is the destruction of the idea that the potency is meant for my enjoyment. The same material energy can be used in the Lord's service, and then the desires for Lord's service, the greatness acquired to serve the Lord, and the entitlement to serve the Lord become sources of perfection. Therefore, two different paths are presented in the Vedic texts. The first path says that to become free of material entanglement, one must destroy the potency or power by curtailing its use; by the cessation of the development of desire, greatness, and entitlement, one can achieve that. The second path says that a more advanced type of perfection can be achieved if we just stop treating this potency or power as something meant for our enjoyment.

The destruction of the chitta is hence different from the purification of the soul's desire. Of course, an impotent man cannot indulge in sex, and he will then lose desire for sex, the pursuit of wealth to get sexual partners, and the entitlement for sex. But a person can also have sex as a service to the Lord, where the desire is to beget spiritually inclined children, great qualities are pursued to find the suitably qualified partner, and there is an entitlement to produce God-conscious children. We will see in later sūtras how this position of this sūtra is modified from the pursuit of impotence to the pursuit of devotion to the Lord. The fact is that most people are not inclined toward God consciousness. If a text begins by saying that you must become the Lord's devotee, then everyone scoffs at the proposal. Hence, the initial discussion is about the soul's suffering in this world, how that suffering can be mitigated by detachment, and how the soul can be liberated from the cycle of birth and death. Once there is enough conviction in a person that such goals are worthy pursuits, instead of the "pursuit of life and happiness", then the superior goal of the pursuit of life and happiness in relationship to the Lord is also presented to the seeker.

Sāñkhya philosophy also describes subsequent manifestations from the ego. These are called the intellect, mind, senses, sensed properties, and sense objects. The sense of entitlement produces a goal, and based on these goals, each person formulates some beliefs. For example, the person who wants to exhibit mastery through money acquires the goal to earn money, and he must have a belief that business, or the stock market, or job employment are good ways to earn money. This belief also transforms into the idea that the world is run by money, and all human relationships are just economic transactions. If someone has the idea of greatness as knowledge, then they may believe that the world can and should be run by ideas, even if it is currently run by wealth. The ideas of greatness are personal, while the beliefs are about the world, how the world works, or how it should work. These beliefs, which are based on the idea of greatness and personal entitlement (which produces goals), are called the intellect, because based on these beliefs we judge if something is true. For example, the person with the idea of wealth as greatness will judge the truth of everything in terms of its economic value. A beautiful theory of nature that cannot be commercialized would not be called great. The person who wants to be great through wealth will instead argue: If this theory were indeed true, then we must be capable of creating some commercial technology from it. Since we are unable to commercialize this scientific theory, therefore it cannot be called true.

Finally, based on the ideas of greatness, the goals, and the beliefs, we create thoughts. For example, the person with the idea of greatness as wealth, the goal of becoming wealthier, and the belief in wealth being the arbiter of truth, will think about how to create more wealth, the changing measures of wealth, how wealth should be protected etc. For him, wealth is right, wealth is good, and wealth is true. These judgments force him to think only of wealth. This is an extreme example to show how the mind works; typically, we have more than one idea of greatness, which makes us evaluate on many dimensions. But if we had only one such idea, then we would think exclusively in these terms.

The recollection of various forms of wealth, whether a person is wealthy in some respect or not, how wealth can be used to decide if some ideas are true or false, etc. rise and fall as waves in an ocean. All these thoughts, intentions, judgments, etc. are manifest from the root—chitta. If the chitta is silenced, for example, during sleep, then it is merely the medium of representation. But when the waves in this medium are produced, e.g., when we wake up and start thinking, intending, judging, desiring, and so on, then the medium is the message.

The silencing of the waves in the chitta is the preliminary goal of yoga, because by its silencing the subsequent stages of ego, intellect, and mind are also quieted. Ultimately, however, we don't have to just silence the chitta; we have to also purify it. What is purification? It is changing the idea of enjoyment. When this desire for enjoyment is changed, then everything else becomes perfect. This ideal will later be defined to be the union with the Supreme Lord. When this idea of greatness is acquired, then the ego is the sense of pride in our relationship to the Lord; the beliefs are the nature of the Supreme Lord; and the thoughts are about the Supreme Lord. The purification of the chitta requires removing the material ideas of enjoyment and replacing them with spiritual enjoyment. If the current ideas remain prominent, then this replacement cannot occur. Therefore, the chitta must be silenced, and if it has been silenced, then naturally new ideas can be acquired. For example, if the chitta is attracted toward money, then a person cannot learn about the Lord. He would always be endeavoring toward earning even more money. Hence, the silencing of the chitta is essential to make spiritual progress, and this is the first step of yoga. But we must remember that this silencing is not the perfection of yoga.

Sūtra 1.3
तदा द्रष्टुःस्वरूपेऽवस्थानम्
tadā draṣṭuḥ svarūpe'vasthānam

tadā—then; draṣṭuḥ—the seer; svarūpe—in one's own form; avasthā-nam—being situated.

TRANSLATION
Then (upon the silencing of the chitta) the seer is situated in its own form.

COMMENTARY
When the chitta becomes active, then thoughts are eventually generated, and the soul's consciousness is directed toward these thoughts. However, when the chitta becomes silent, then there is no content to be aware of. In this situation, the soul becomes prominently aware of its own existence as the seer of all these things. In fact, the soul now sees itself to be distinct from the thoughts.

This is important because in the materially conditioned state, the soul doesn't even realize how it is different from the body and the mind. When the soul identifies itself with the body and the mind, then it doesn't believe that it has free will—because it is dragged by the wants and needs of the body and the mind. If the soul is not seen to be different from the body and the mind, then the questions of a transcendental experience do not arise. The material reality is considered the only reality, and the self is seen to be just the body and the mind. To pursue transcendental experience, one must know that he is not the body and the mind, and this can be realized when the mind and the body are completely calmed, and yet, the soul is fully conscious. In short, there can be self-consciousness without a thought, a feeling, a judgment, or an intention. But to realize this fact, one must make the body and the mind totally calm.

When the body and the mind are calmed, then the soul realizes its power over the body and the mind, and that power is understood to be the free will. The will is simply that the soul can engage with the experience of the body and the mind, or be completely disengaged from it. Since one can go from the state of disengagement to engagement, and vice versa, the material mind and the body cannot be causes of free will. The soul is now seen to be transcendent to the body and the mind, and we ask: Who am I, if not the body and the mind?

Sūtra 1.4
वृत्तसिारूप्यमतिरत्र
vṛttisārūpyamitaratra

vṛtti—the modifications; sārūpyam—being one with; itaratra—being other.

TRANSLATION
Being one with the modification (of the chitta) is being other than the self.

COMMENTARY
A consequence of the silencing of the mind is that the self is dissociated with the material thoughts, feelings, judgments, and intentions. One realizes that their consciousness can be withdrawn from these and focused on the soul's interest. When this control over thoughts, feelings, judgments, and intentions is obtained, then the soul is seen as the master, and everything else is seen as something that the master can employ, and yet, not be controlled by them.

When you observe a flower, and are absorbed in admiring that flower, then momentarily you forget your existence. You lose the sense that my experience is *about* the flower, and the self is different from the flower. In other words, there is flower-consciousness, without the self-consciousness. You are effectively 'lost' in the experience of the flower. Similarly, when the soul observes the body, it loses the self-consciousness, being fully absorbed in body-consciousness. Of course, the self can observe the body dispassionately and retain the self-consciousness. In that state, our experience would be *about* the body, without losing the self-awareness.

Thus, there are two distinct ways in which our ordinary experiences exist. In the first, experience has 'aboutness' which comes with self-awareness, and in the second, it doesn't. There is no harm in saying that my experience is 'about' my mind and body, which means that I can see it, but it is not me—the self is distinct from the body. The problem of bodily identity begins when this 'aboutness' is lost. Then we don't say that my experience is 'about' the body and the mind; we say: "I am thinking", "I am feeling", etc. rather than "I see a thought", "I see a feeling". Due to this fact, the materialistic philosopher claims that there is no difference between the soul and the body, because they don't have a developed consciousness which observes even the body and the mind dispassionately, as if it were an act in a theatre.

Thus, this sūtra notes that when this aboutness of experience is lost, then we lose the sense that we are distinct from the body and mind, and that situation is comparable to our looking at a flower and being so lost in that perception such that we forget our individuality separate from the flower. The preliminary liberation from the body and the mind is when we can observe the body and the mind, while remaining aware of our separate identity. If we detach ourselves from the body and the mind, then we find that the thoughts, feelings, intentions, judgments, etc. cease. Merely restoring the aboutness of our consciousness in relation to the body and the mind totally silences the chitta.

Sūtra 1.5

वृत्तयःपञ्चतय्यःक्लिष्टा अक्लिष्टाः

vṛttayaḥ pañcatayyaḥ kliṣṭā akliṣṭāḥ

vṛttayaḥ—the modifications of the chitta; pañcatayyaḥ—are five-fold; kliṣṭāḥ—those that are painful; akliṣṭāḥ—those that are painless.

TRANSLATION

The modifications of the chitta are five-fold; they are painful and painless.

COMMENTARY

These five-fold modifications are described in the next sūtra. This exact sūtra also occurs in Sāṅkhya Sūtras as the sūtra 2.33. However, in the

Sāṅkhya Sūtras, these five modifications are said to be the modifications of the 'dhī' or the intellect. From this, we must understand that these are the five states of each of the internal instruments, namely, the chitta, mahattattva (the ideas about greatness), ego (the entitlement), intellect (beliefs), and the mind (thoughts).

Sūtra 1.6
प्रमाणवपिर्ययवकिल्पनद्रिास्मृतयः
pramāṇaviparyayavikalpanidrāsmṛtayaḥ

pramāṇa—correct knowledge; viparyaya—opposite (incorrect knowledge); vikalpa—doubt; nidrā—deep sleep; and smṛti—memory (are the five modifications).

TRANSLATION

Correct knowledge, incorrect knowledge, doubt, deep sleep, and memory (are the five modifications of the chitta).

COMMENTARY

Deep sleep is the primordial state of the chitta, in which it remains silent. Then, in the memory state, the impressions and the knowledge acquired in the past manifest as thoughts. Thoughts can also arise due to the interaction with the external world, and the mental aspect of the chitta is activated to understand the external world. Either due to internal modification of the chitta, or due to its external triggering, the resulting thoughts often have inconsistencies. For example, we might wonder if the thing we are seeing is a horse or a zebra. Similarly, two thoughts might arise simultaneously—one that said that we should eat something, and the other that says that eating too much is harmful to our health. Due to the inconsistencies in the various appearing thoughts, a doubt arises, which is the conflicted state of the chitta. This conflict is resolved when one of the thoughts is prioritized. This prioritization may reject either the correct or the incorrect thought, which in turn leads to incorrect and correct knowledge. When the correct knowledge is attained, the chitta remains stable as we are confident about our perception. However, if the incorrect knowledge is attained, the chitta remains disturbed, because there are doubts and guilt about the prioritization. Of course, if we don't know what correct and incorrect knowledge is, then we can remain quite peaceful even under the incorrect judgment. But if incorrect idea is prioritized knowingly, then the chitta remains disturbed. The 'truth' and 'falsity' of the thought are part of the chitta in the sense that we strongly believe in some ideas, and believe less strongly in others. These beliefs can be changed, and they are often changed due to incompatibility with other beliefs—because we seek the greatest amount of peace and tranquility and inconsistencies in the thoughts keeps the chitta disturbed. Thus, when we encounter two beliefs that are mutually incompatible, sometimes we choose in favor of what we believe to be true. However, if that true belief isn't working, then the belief is weakened by doubt, and then the false belief may be chosen as an alternative under the conjecture that our belief could be wrong. In this way, the working of the chitta can be understood through these five states.

<h2 style="text-align:center">Sūtra 1.7</h2>

प्रत्यक्षानुमानागमाःप्रमाणानि
pratyakṣānumānāgamāḥ pramāṇāni

pratyakṣa—direct observation; anumāna—inference; āgama—scriptural evidence; pramāṇāni—are the methods of evidence or proof.

<h3 style="text-align:center">TRANSLATION</h3>

Direct observation, inference, and scriptural evidence are the methods of evidence or proof.

<h3 style="text-align:center">COMMENTARY</h3>

Direct observation includes not just sense perception but even mental perception (the mind is considered the sixth sense in Sāṅkhya), and even experience of the soul. Ultimately, the soul's experience is the final evidence, so, pratyakṣa is very important, if we include the soul's experience within it. This true pratyakṣa involves the clear separation between the various tiers of perception such as sensation, thought, judgment, intention, values, and the self. If these things are not clearly separated, then the 'aboutness' of experience is missing, and it is not truly pratyakṣa because we are not seeing everything.

As far as the experience of the five senses is concerned, there are two doctrines that must be considered—verification and falsification. The problem with verification is that just because we have observed something many times, we cannot conclude it to be true, because it may not be observed subsequently. To overcome this problem, direct observation is used only as a method of falsification—even if we observe the truth to not be confirmed by observation once (assuming that observation was carried out correctly), it is not considered true. However, if direct perception is extended to all the possible faculties, including consciousness, then direct perception can also be used for verification because then we can see deeper levels of reality that we cannot see by the five senses.

Since we cannot see many things by the five senses, therefore, inferences can be used to interpret the sense observations. The purpose of an inference is to guess the nature of the reality that we could not perceive. However, since all inferences involve some guesswork, therefore, they are inherently unreliable. Also, the same sense perception can be interpreted in more than one way. Again, to overcome this problem, we can use falsification instead of verification. For instance, we can say that if some inference cannot be used to explain some sense observation even once, then that inference must be considered falsified.

Thus, if we speak of sense observation and mental inference as methods of proof, they are more correctly methods of falsification rather than verification. This issue arises due to the inherent limitations of the senses and the mind.

The spiritual experience is a method of verification, but its absence is not a method of falsification. For example, if the soul has acquired the capacity for direct perception, then the capacity can be used for verification. However, if someone hasn't developed a spiritual capacity for perception, then their inability to perceive cannot be considered falsification of spiritual experience.

Vedic scriptural evidence, however, can be used both for falsification and verification. If some statements are found in a Vedic scripture, then they can be considered true—and we can verify them by sense observation and inference. Likewise, if some claims contradict the scriptural statements, then they can be considered false—and we can confirm this by inference and observation. The verification of scriptural evidence can also be achieved by spiritual experience. Likewise, the falsification of statements contrary to Vedic scriptures can also be confirmed by spiritual experience. Thus, the Vedic scriptures become authoritative because their claims can always be confirmed through observation.

In one sense, each of these methods are complete. If we can obtain all the observations, or study all the scriptures, or reason about all the problems, then we can use these methods individually to determine the truth. But if one of these are not present, then we can use the other methods as complements. For example, in lieu of direct observation, we can use reasoning or scriptural statements to provisionally accept the truth, while we pursue direct experience.

Sūtra 1.8
विपर्ययो मिथ्याज्ञानमतद्रूपप्रतिष्ठम्
viparyayo mithyājñānamatadrūpapratiṣṭham

viparyayaḥ—the opposites; mithyā—false; jñānam—knowledge; atadrūpa—mistaken ideas about a thing's nature; pratiṣṭham—it is established.

TRANSLATION
It is established that the opposite methods produce false knowledge, creating mistaken ideas about a thing's nature.

COMMENTARY
A good example of an alternative method for ascertaining the truth is popularity of an idea. This method is widely employed at present, where people consider something to be true simply because many people accept it. Most people who go by the popularity of that thing don't ask: Is this idea rational? Has it been proven empirically? Is there scriptural evidence for its truth? They just think that if many people believe in something, then *they* must have performed these tests. Thus, false ideas come into fashion and go out of fashion, and what is considered true today is considered false tomorrow. The reason is that it has not been proven rationally, confirmed empirically, or stated by scriptures.

Similarly, people may believe in irrational ideas, those that are not substantiated by empirical evidence, and those that are contrary to the scriptural statements. Many rational ideas that are not empirically substantiated are also false. Likewise, many empirical observations that are not backed by rational analysis may merely be hallucinations or visual illusions. Finally, even those things that seem rational and empirical in a smaller domain may be false when we extend the domain to a wider variety of phenomena. The scriptural truth is that which applies to everything; this is not merely because it is stated in the scripture, but can also be tested empirically and verified rationally. If one doesn't believe in the scripture, then they can try to extend their empirical and rational claims to other domains and they will find that they become inapplicable or false upon that extension. The scriptural truth, on the other hand, doesn't become false even when it is extended to the entire existence. The doubters about the scriptural truth can confirm this by extending the scriptural ideas to all subjects and domains. The Vedic system therefore asserts that even many empirical and rational claims that are limited to a small domain are not true unless they accord with the scriptural truth. This is not a blind faith in the scriptures; it is based on the fact that enlightened souls have found its applicability to all domains.

Sūtra 1.9
शब्दज्ञानानुपाती वस्तुशून्यो विकल्पः
śabdajñānānupātī vastuśūnyo vikalpaḥ

śabda—the scriptural; jñāna—knowledge; anupātī—follows as a consequence; vastu—a real thing; śūnyaḥ—absence of; vikalpa—alternatives.

TRANSLATION
The scriptural knowledge follows as a consequence of a real thing, and the absence of alternatives.

COMMENTARY
The scriptural evidence is produced by an authoritative personality after the direct observation of something, along with the careful rational consideration of why the alternative cannot be true. In short, scriptural evidence is also the application of direct observation and inference, although by an enlightened soul. We can liken this type of evidence to the testimony given by experts in a field. For example, if an expert doctor gives an opinion about something, based on his decades of direct observation, and a careful rational analysis of why the alternative cannot be true, then that opinion is considered to be true. Of course, ordinary humans have many faults, and they can commit mistakes. The true scriptural evidence is that which is presented by the faultless personality. The faultiness of the author can be established if

any of their statements are proven to be false. However, if they are always proven true, by the method prescribed for confirming them, then the fault-lessness of the author is established. Then, we can take their other statements to be true based on their established authority, although every such statement must be confirmed by reason and observation. Faith thus has a role in getting us jumpstarted in acquiring knowledge: We can learn from the authorities and then confirm it by their given method.

Sūtra 1.10
अभावपरत्ययालम्बना वृत्तिर्निदिरा
abhāvapratyayālambanā vṛttirnidrā

abhāva—absence; pratyaya—the intelligence; ālambanā—support of; vṛttiḥ—the modification; nidrā—called deep sleep.

TRANSLATION
(The proof by) absence is based on the support of the deep sleep modification of the intelligence.

COMMENTARY
Some schools of Vedic philosophy (e.g., Nyāya) accept absence as a method of proof. This method can be applied both with inference and observation. In the case of inference, this is called proof by contradiction, but the problem is that many seeming contradictions have been resolved by introducing new ways of thinking, so the proof by contradiction is not always considered a valid method. Similarly, there are situations in which we cannot resolve these contradictions because we don't have the new ideas, so they *seem* like contradictions although they are not. For example, atomic theory uses contradictory ideas of 'wave' and 'particle' to describe quanta. In one sense, we have a new idea that reconciles the previously disparate theories of light and matter, so waves and particles are no longer contradictory. In another sense, we don't truly understand what can simultaneously be a wave and a particle, so they are indeed contradictory. This ability to introduce new ideas, and use them to resolve contradictions is pretty standard in the history of science and philosophy, so what seems like a contradiction may not truly be contradictory, and hence proof by contradiction is not a perfect method to knowledge. Likewise, in the

case of observation, observing absence is equivalent to not observing the intended object, but that non-observation could also be attributed to the absence of the correct method of observation. If we don't see the sun some-day, because the sky is cloudy, we cannot conclude that the sun has ceased to exist. Therefore, observation of absence is not the confirmation of the absence itself. As the popular statement asserts: "Absence of evidence is not evidence of absence".

This sūtra states that non-observation is found even during sleeping, so how can we use it to conclude that something indeed is absent? The point is that due to faulty reasoning and imperfect senses, we may not perceive something (or even its effects). In Sāṅkhya, reality also exists as a potential, so its observation requires a process by which that potential manifests into a reality. Material reality is also eternal in Sāṅkhya, so everything that can ever exist, exists right now potentially (or in a manifested state). We may not be able to see that potential or reality, but that doesn't mean it doesn't exist. It may be invisible to us because we did not follow the correct pro-cedure of observation. Given the eternity of all possibilities, the absence of observation is compared to the sleeping state; the potential for observation exists, but it is not observed.

Sūtra 1.11
अनुभूतवषियासम्प्रमोषःस्मृतिः
anubhūtaviṣayāsampramoṣaḥ smṛtiḥ

anubhūta—experienced; viṣaya—in the subject; asampramoṣaḥ—with-out any loss; smṛti—are the smṛti scriptures.

TRANSLATION
Experienced in the subject, without any loss, are the smṛti scriptures.

COMMENTARY
In the earlier sūtra, the āgama were mentioned as scriptures. This sūtra mentions an even broader category of scriptures called the smṛti, which include the Purana, Tantra (which are called āgama), histories such as Ramayana and the Mahabharata, etc. The śruti are always accepted to be evidences, but some people challenge the authorities of the smṛti, stating that these are subsequent to the śruti, so perhaps somehow inferior to

them. This sūtra counters such conjectures and states that the smṛti are equally well-versed in the subject, and they do not omit anything that is already present in the śrutī. The difference is that the style of presentation in smṛti is conversational, whereas the style of presentation in the śrutī can sometimes be aphoristic, concise, or terse. The differences in the styles of presentation do not entail a difference in the truth of their claims, or the validity of the knowledge that they are presenting in a narrative style.

Sūtra 1.12
अभ्यासवैराग्याभ्यां तन्निरोधः
abhyāsavairāgyābhyāṁ tannirodhaḥ

abhyāsa—practice; vairāgyābhyām—and by detachment; tat—those (modifications of the chitta); nirodhaḥ—are suppressed.

TRANSLATION
By practice and detachment, those (modifications of the chitta) are suppressed.

COMMENTARY
Detachment plays an extremely important role in spiritual life because unless a person is detached from materialistic endeavors, there is no progress. We can liken the spiritual activities of a materially attached person to a man rowing a boat tied to the shore. Even as one practices spiritual life, their mind is always thinking about mundane things. For example, if a person deeply attached to his family, profession, or material possessions sits for meditation, his awareness is distracted to other attachments. Even as meditation is performed, it doesn't produce the expected results—just as one might row a boat tied to the shore.

Conversely, when a person becomes detached from his materialistic endeavors, then their meditation is indeed effective, because the mind is engaged in that activity, rather than being distracted by a thousand different ideas and priorities. A materially attached person might think that they are doing justice to both material and spiritual activities, but they do not make spiritual progress, such as obtaining realization of how the body is different from the soul. Hence, as the practice of yoga acquaints us with a new reality that we haven't earlier seen, to truly progress on this path, one must also practice detachment.

Sūtra 1.13
तत्र स्थितौ यत्नोऽभ्यासः
tatra sthitau yatno'bhyāsaḥ

tatra—there; sthitau—situated; yatnaḥ—effort; abhyāsah—practice.

TRANSLATION
By practice and effort, there (in a detached mental state) situated.

COMMENTARY
The statements about practice have been made earlier, but in the previous sūtra, detachment was emphasized along with practice. There is no other way to obtain detachment, other than to practice it. For example, while performing meditation one must be able to focus the mind exclusively on that activity. If the mind is distracted into other things, then it is not considered meditation. This generally means performing meditation in the early hours, when the mind is quiet. The practice of detachment also means always giving a higher priority to spiritual activities, and delegating all other activities to a time *after* the spiritual activities have been performed. Typically, most people practice yoga in their 'free time'—after all the material activities have been completed. In this situation, yoga remains a hobby, a pastime, akin to entertainment, which we indulge in after life's priorities are completed. With that attitude, however, there is very little earnestness and hence little gain. For example, if you were painting as a hobby, it doesn't matter if the picture doesn't come out perfect. If you were practicing music as a hobby, it doesn't matter if you take a long time to learn an instrument. Indeed, in most cases, there is no desire for obtaining perfection in our hobbies. There are feeble goals, there is no urgency, and nothing is believed to have been lost if these are unattained. If spiritual life is pursued with that attitude, then the results of that practice are proportional.

Therefore, it is important to understand that perfection comes when spiritual life becomes the primary—if not the only goal—in a person's life. And this requires detachment from every other goal that we were previously engaged in. When we begin practicing detachment, we find that we are always pulled back to the ordinary life, and the focus is lost. The sincere practitioner, however, puts in greater effort now to reprioritize and refocus on spiritual activities. By repeated return to the primary focus, a person gradually attains a state where he is either never distracted, or even if some emergencies are to be attended to, they are disposed minimally and swiftly, and focus returns to spirituality. This process can be long-drawn, but this sūtra says that it is always attainable.

Sūtra 1.14
स तु दीर्घकालनैरन्तर्यसत्कारासेवितो दृढभूमिः
sa tu dīrghakālanairantaryasatkārāsevito dṛḍhabhūmiḥ

saḥ—he (the materially conditioned soul); tu—but; dīrghakāla—a long time; nairantarya—without interruption; satkāra—the eternal activity; asevito—not serving; dṛḍhabhūmiḥ—solid earth.

TRANSLATION
He (the materially conditioned soul) is but a solid earth due to not serving the eternal activity uninterrupted for a long time.

COMMENTARY
The material conditioning is very hard, and very difficult to give up. We have been identifying with the body, indulging in materialistic activities for very long. Life after life we have identified with the body, its associates, its survival, and its enjoyment. Due to this prolonged habit of serving the body and its interests, there is no realization about how the soul is different from the body. Whatever the body and the mind generate as needs and wants, the soul simply agrees to fulfill them. In this situation, this sūtra warns, the cessation of thoughts in the chitta also takes a long time. Just like digging solid earth is very hard, and it takes a long time, similarly, progress is elongated due to the fixed nature of our attachments and habits. After stating that perfection can be attained, a warning is also presented—don't expect it to happen very quickly. If you persist, it is attainable, but constant endeavor and persistence is needed.

Sūtra 1.15
दृष्टानुश्रवकिवषियवतृष्णस्य वशीकारसज्ज्ञा वैराग्यम्
dṛṣṭānuśravikaviṣayavitṛṣṇasya vaśīkārasañjñā vairāgyam

dṛṣṭa—the seer; ānuśravika—repeatedly hearing; viṣaya—the objects of sense enjoyment; vitṛṣṇasya—devoid of the lust for; vaśīkāra—brings under control; sañjñā—is called; vairāgyam—detachment.

TRANSLATION

The seer, by repeatedly hearing, becomes devoid of the lust for the objects of sense enjoyment, and brings under control (his lust); this is called detachment.

COMMENTARY

The discussion on detachment is continued in this sūtra, which emphasizes the process of repeated hearing. What is this hearing? It is the hearing about the futility of material life. If we are successful in material endeavors, then we repeat the cycle of birth and death. And if we fail in material endeavors, then we become unhappy. This is not a win-win, or win-lose situation; it is a lose-lose situation. Both success and failure in material endeavors increase the bondage. When one repeatedly hears about the futility of material endeavors, and takes it seriously, then gradually he gives up the outward-bound focus of the senses and the mind—that are always chasing the pleasure of the body—and withdraws inward into the true self-interest. This disengagement from the lust for material things, relationships, and sense pleasure is called detachment.

Sūtra 1.16
तत्परं पुरुषख्यातेर्गुणवैतृष्ण्यम्
tatparaṁ puruṣakhyāterguṇavaitṛṣṇyam

tatparaṁ—thereafter; puruṣa—the soul; khyāteḥ—reputation is known; guṇa—the material qualities; vaitṛṣṇyam—devoid of the lust.

TRANSLATION

Thereafter, the soul's reputation is known as devoid of the lust for material qualities.

COMMENTARY

The soul is great, beautiful, and eternal. It has infinite abilities which lie undiscovered. It has immense power by which it can accomplish great things. But this great, beautiful, and eternal soul has presently become a servant of the body, where he serves a master that is not great, not beautiful, and not eternal. But we cannot know the nature of the great, beautiful, and eternal soul unless we become free of material lust—i.e., stop serving the not great, not beautiful, and not eternal master. Liberation doesn't mean getting out of this body, because after this body there will be another body. Liberation simply means becoming the master of this body, and using it for the purpose of the soul. Why should something great, beautiful, and eternal serve the much inferior? The problem is that we don't know how eternally great and beautiful the soul is. So, we have accepted an inferior position of serving the bodily needs and wants. If these needs and wants are brought under control, then the soul is realized. This sūtra calls this knowledge the 'reputation' of the soul. This reputation comes from the Vedic scriptures where the soul is described as being unbreakable, full of happiness, and capable of unprecedented things. Conditioned by the body, the same soul is forced into mediocrity, suffering, and repeated birth and death. So, we should, in our interest, get out of the clutches of this entanglement.

Sūtra 1.17

वतिर्कवचिारानन्दास्मतिारूपानुगमात्सम्परज्ञातः

vitarkavicārānandāsmitārūpānugamātsamprajñātaḥ

vitarka—argument; vicāra—thought; ānanda—enjoyment; asmitā—egotism; rūpa—the form; anugamāt—by approaching; samprajñātaḥ—is called balanced intelligence.

TRANSLATION

By approaching (i.e., trying to understand) the form (of the soul) by argument, thought, enjoyment, and egotism, is called balanced intelligence.

COMMENTARY

There are many ways to understand the nature of the soul, and this sūtra notes four such methods. The method of argument can go as follows. In this life, the soul has a childhood body, a youthful body, and an old body. Through all these bodies, the identity of the person remains unchanged. How can that identity be unchanged when the body is constantly changing? Naturally, that identity has to be assigned to something that is different from the body. Similarly, if someone has committed a crime a few years ago, we don't say that the body has changed, so the person is different, and therefore, the new body should not be punished. Rather, the new body is punished, because the person is still the same. Likewise, if someone has borrowed money from a bank in the past, we don't say that the body has changed, so the person must have changed, and therefore, there is no need to repay the loan. We rather insist that the same person borrowed the loan, so they have to repay it. In this way, even in this life, the person's identity persists despite the bodily changes, so that identity must be assigned to something that is not the body, and that must be the soul.

The argument from thought can go as follows. Thoughts automatically arise in our mind, and we have the choice to focus on the thought, or reject it. We can give up our past bad habits, and acquire new habits. We can change our ways of thinking, alter our beliefs, and even modify our goals. The possibility of all such changes points to the necessity of choice, which is different from the thoughts, judgments, intentions, and beliefs. Since each of these can be accepted or rejected, therefore, the mechanism of accepting or rejecting them must be different from the content of experience which is accepted or rejected. Therefore, the entity that makes the choice must be different from the content.

The argument from enjoyment can go as follows. Nobody wants to suffer, but the suffering comes anyway. Why is it that we all want to be happy, but the happiness is not available to us? Why is there so much suffering in the world? Indeed, why is there so much discrepancy in the pleasures afforded to different people? Why are some people rich, while others are poor? Why are some people healthy while others are sick? The rational response to these questions is that there is a soul which has performed misdeeds, and it is consequently forced to suffer in different ways. That also means that the soul is eternal and not restricted to this body. Then, if the soul learns the art and science of moral actions, then it can become free of this suffering. Indeed, it can be situated in the self even while material suffering is going on, and minimize the resulting pain. Thus, by under-standing the cause and mitigation of suffering, the soul is established. If one doesn't accept the soul, however, then he goes on suffering.

The argument from egotism can go as follows. What is my true self-interest? I have been serving ungrateful people in this life, and despite being sincere toward my responsibilities, they don't treat me with respect. Rather, they see me as an instrument for their happiness. Therefore, instead of serving the selfish people blindly, and hoping for reciprocation, I must look at my self-interest. What is that self-interest? Obviously, we can live completely alone, but that will not be very pleasing. Our true self-interest is that we live with truly kind, gracious, and unselfish people who recip-rocate our love with greater love. Who are these people? They are the ones who have realized their difference from the body. They are free from fear, greed, and lust, and they are always kind, compassionate, and gracious. If I want to be happy, therefore, I must also become just like them because then I don't have to live in the company of ungrateful and entitled people, and I can associate only with the enlightened souls.

In this way, one can convince oneself of the importance of spiritual life, and become detached. If detachment from the material conditions is obtained, then there is natural attachment to transcendence, since the soul cannot remain idle and purposeless. It always seeks the purpose of exis-tence, but if the purpose is materialistic, then true happiness and knowl-edge are never obtained. Hence, it is very important to convince ourselves to become detached from the sources of incessant suffering and focus on the sources of permanent happiness.

Sūtra 1.18

वरिामप्रत्ययाभ्यासपूरव:संस्कारशेषोऽन्यः

virāmapratyayābhyāsapūrvaḥ saṁskāraśeṣo'nyaḥ

virāma—the cessation; pratyaya—needs and wants; abhyāsa—the practice; pūrvaḥ—as stated before; saṁskāra—the habits and impressions; śeṣaḥ—end or terminate; anyaḥ—the other.

TRANSLATION

By the practice, as stated before, there is cessation of all other (i.e., not related to yoga) needs and wants, the habits and impressions of the past.

COMMENTARY

The previous sūtras noted that by repeated hearing and practice, by argument, by thought, by understanding the true nature of suffering and its effects, and by focusing on the self-interest, one must obtain detachment. This sūtra says that if we follow all these methods, then one becomes detached from the needs and wants, the habits and impressions acquired over previous lives. We can call this process of 'hearing' about the futility of material life as the preliminary step toward the performance of yoga. In the previous sūtras, the true nature of the soul was described as being beyond the body. However, most people are preoccupied with the needs and wants of the body, and spend most of their life just protecting, feeding, and sustaining their body in the hope that they will enjoy with it. The price they incur for this enjoyment is immense, and the enjoyment is always temporary. Under the ignorance about the soul, and how its enjoyment is continuous, and has zero cost, they keep focusing on temporary pleasures that cost a lot. This type of pleasure is therefore considered ignorance, however, unless one knows about the soul, bodily pleasure remains the only imaginable source of happiness. To detach us out of this cycle of suffering and enjoying, one has to 'hear' about the true nature of material existence, and then convince oneself of its futility by argument, thought, enjoyment, and egotism as described in the previous sūtra. If this process of detachment is followed correctly, then, this sūtra states, one becomes free of the inexorable pull of material lust. That freedom is the termination of false impressions and habits.

Sūtra 1.19

भवप्रत्ययो वदिेहप्रकृतिलयानाम्

bhavapratyayo videhaprakṛtilayānām

bhava—being; pratyayah—the desires and wants; videha—free of the body; prakṛti—modes of nature; layānām—the merger. .

TRANSLATION

Being free of the body of desires and wants, the merger of modes of nature.

COMMENTARY

In Sāṅkhya philosophy, beyond the gross body that we can perceive, the gendered body of mind, intellect, ego, and the moral sense, there is another deeper body of desires and habits called the subtle body. It is an aspect of the body that is identified as the chitta and sometimes called the body of impressions. The soul is automatically controlled by this body because desires and thoughts automatically spring from the body of impressions and habits. As the soul acts on these desires and impressions, the subtle body is further reinforced, and the same desires and impressions perpetuate. These impressions are described to have three kinds of qualities of prakṛti called sattva, rajas, and tamas.

In tamas, we are always unhappy and depressed; we see the world cynically, and even if some happiness is derived, it is through sarcasm, irony, or mockery. At best, tamas is the enjoyment of the absurdity of the world—which may include the absurdity of our own lives, or those of other people around us. And at worst, tamas is the anger and frustration caused by the hopeless situations. In rajas, we are sometimes happy and sometimes unhappy. This is a life lived in pursuit of material results, and we are happy if they are obtained and unhappy if they are not. And in sattva, we are peaceful and satisfied, and we remain equanimous to all situations. Due to sattva, a person is interested in true knowledge. Due to rajas, one is impelled toward materialistic achievement and enjoyment in this world. And due to tamas, the soul relinquishes material duties, becomes lazy, and sometimes even loses a sense of purpose in life.

The spiritual state is beyond the three modes, and it is considered the 'merger' of the three modes. The merger indicates that the soul has knowledge of its true nature, is always enjoying within itself, and becomes materially inert due to relinquishment of worldly purposes. The inertness seems just like tamas, but it is not material laziness; it is complete disengagement with worldly purposes. The desire for pleasure seems just like rajas, but it is not passion for worldly achievements; it is the enjoyment of inner bliss. Finally, the true knowledge doesn't pertain to the nature of the external world, but to the self; the inertness and passion are not delusional; they are caused by truly knowing the self.

The material world separates these three modes. As a result, those truly interested in knowledge are not lazy and not interested in worldly name, fame, love, and achievement; just the knowledge of the truth is a reward in itself. Those truly interested in name, fame, love, and achievement are not truly interested in the nature of the truth, and they are not lazy either. As long as they get success, they don't care about the truth. Finally, the lazy and inert are neither interested in the nature of the truth, nor in worldly achievements. They just enjoy not working hard and not thinking about the nature of the truth. Thus, sattva, rajas, and tamas are separated by their qualities in the material world. And the soul, which is transcendent to the material world, combines these three qualities. There is hence the appearance of laziness, passion, and knowledge in the enlightened soul, and the contradictions between the qualities disappears. The perfected soul acquires all the goodness of the three qualities, and loses all the disadvantages of these qualities. This combination is called perfection.

This sūtra states that this perfection of the combination of the three qualities is acquired when one becomes free of material needs and wants. In this freedom, there is true knowledge of the self, enjoyment of the self, and outward inertness and disinterest from worldly aspirations. Therefore, the perfected soul is not free of qualities; it is rather free of the separated material qualities.

Becoming free from material desires doesn't mean the end of the soul's native desires for spiritual happiness. The soul is capable of generating happiness, making others happy, because it is happy by itself, and that happiness is not due to a reason—e.g., that I'm happy because I have obtained this or that material object. This happiness is causeless; it exists automatically. However, we have forgotten that natural state of happiness, and we have started considering the needs and wants of this body as the cause of happiness. Thus, if the body is fed and satisfied, then we are happy; otherwise not. Once we get past this materialistic idea of happiness, then we realize that the soul is automatically happy. This is freedom from the body. It doesn't mean death of the body. It means that regardless of the condition of the body we are always happy.

In this state of happiness, there is still a desire. But it is not a desire of taking something to become happy. It is the desire to spread real happiness by giving others spiritual knowledge without the expectation of a return. Thus, a progressive realization is described in these sūtras where one first obtains detachment, then realizes the nature of the self, and then becomes imbued with a new kind of qualities, which are different from the previous material qualities. The impersonal philosopher thinks that liberation is freedom from all qualities. But he doesn't realize that the soul has its own qualities. When the material qualities are rejected, then the true qualities of the soul gradually become visible.

Sūtra 1.20
श्रद्धावीर्यस्मृतिसिमाधिप्रज्ञापूर्वक इतरेषाम्
śraddhāvīryasmṛtisamādhiprajñāpūrvaka itareṣām

śraddhā—trust; vīrya—vigor; smṛti—memory; samādhī—being the same as the origin; prajñāpūrvaka—with full cognition; itareṣām—this other is called.

TRANSLATION

Trust, vigor, memory, (are spiritual qualities) and prajñāpūrvaka-samādhī is having them, or being like the origin of everything with full cognition.

COMMENTARY

The origin of everything is the Supreme Lord, and He is full of spiritual qualities. When the soul attains perfection, he also become just like the Lord. This sūtra describes three qualities of this state—trust, vigor, and memory.

What is trust? It doesn't mean mere faith in the guru or scriptures. It is rather the state free of doubts. It is also a state in which the self-doubts—e.g., about our capacity to understand the nature of the truth or practice the truth—are destroyed. Hence, trust also means 'self-confidence' in the sense that we are no longer considered incapable of understanding and practicing the spiritual truth. This brings freedom from fear and uncertainty—the fear that I will fail in spiritual endeavors, and the uncertainty that the results of such endeavors may not fructify to the extent that I want them to. Hence, 'trust' is a broad category of spiritual qualities of fearlessness, confidence, and destruction of doubts.

What is vigor? It doesn't mean physical strength; we are talking about spiritual rather than material qualities. As a spiritual quality it represents that inner vitality because of which one is never bored, tired, weak, or devoid of excitedness. Rather, one is always enthusiastic. In that enthusiastic state, there is constant pursuit of unchartered territories, zeal for spiritual exploration, and the discovery of novelty. Vigor or vitality is hence a spiritual quality that leads a person to constantly endeavor toward greater self-realization, the service of the Lord, and the efforts to mitigate the conditions of those who are suffering.

What is memory? It represents the absence of forgetfulness of our own nature, of the nature of the world, and the nature of the Supreme Lord. With this constant remembrance, the soul becomes flawless, and doesn't commit mistakes, because he is fully aware of the consequences of all his activities.

So, these terms—trust, vigor, and memory—should be understood by contrasting them to the material state in which we are full of fear and doubts, weakness and boredom, ignorance and forgetfulness. Liberation from the material condition doesn't mean mere withdrawal from the body and the mind, or the engagement with the world. It is rather the discovery of the self. Now one might think that the realization of the self would be just the cognition of the self as different from the body. While that is indeed part of the truth, it is only the initial stage. When the self is recognized different from the body, we also discover infinite vitality, vigor, freedom from fear, and full knowledge. So, this is the true goal of yoga, namely, the discovery of the greatness of the soul.

Sūtra 1.21
तीव्रसंवेगानामासन्नः
tīvrasaṁvegānāmāsannaḥ

tīvra—intense; saṁvegānām—excited intensity; āsannaḥ—fulfilment.

TRANSLATION
(The perfected state) is intense, excited intensity, and fulfilment.

COMMENTARY
Many people consider detachment from the material world to be the end of all joy and happiness. They think that if we give up the material enjoyment, then life would be so boring and placid. This sūtra instead states that once the true nature of the soul is discovered, there is constant excitement. There is never a dull or boring moment because fulfillment, joy, and excitement come from within. There is no cause for this excitement and intensity. It is spontaneous and causeless. The spiritually advanced

person doesn't need material achievements, name, fame, and followers, power, wealth, or recognition, to be happy. He is happy for no ostensible reason. He is ever fulfilled and totally satisfied. In fact, he is so excited in his condition, that he is ever willing to spread happiness. This inner state of spontaneous joy is the very nature of the enlightened soul.

Sūtra 1.22
मृदुमध्याधिमात्रत्वात्ततोऽपि विशेषः
mṛdumadhyādhimātratvāttato'pi viśeṣaḥ

mṛdu—soft; madhya—moderate; adhimātratvāt—due to being as if above all measures; api—even (in this case also); viśeṣaḥ—are the qualities.

TRANSLATION
Softness and moderation, due to being as if above all measures, are even (in this case also) the qualities (of the soul).

COMMENTARY
The impersonal philosopher says that the soul is not hard or soft, not moderate or excessive, but this sūtra differs. It says that the liberated condition makes the person very soft, compassionate, accommodating. But that doesn't mean that he also accepts nonsense as truth. Therefore, he is also considered moderate—i.e., sometimes soft, and sometimes hard. In this way, the perfected soul is beyond all ordinary measures, beyond ordinary classifications and categorizations of persons. The use of the term viśeṣa means that the soul has qualities. But these qualities are different from material qualities because in the material world, if something is soft then it is not hard and if something is hard, then it is not soft. Material nature gives us a fixed personality, by which we can classify a person into a personality type. But spiritual nature is different; it cannot be classified and categorized according to the material classes and categories because it accepts the truth and rejects the falsity; it tolerates personal inconveniences and fights the ignorance and mistruths. The perfect soul is not bound by the designations or compelled to behave in a predetermined manner. So, he is beyond the material qualities, but not devoid of qualities themselves.

Sūtra 1.23
ईश्वरप्रणिधानाद्वा
īśvarapraṇidhānādvā

īśvara—the Lord; praṇidhānāt—due to surrender and devotion; vā—alternatively.

TRANSLATION

Alternatively, due to surrender and devotion to the Lord (the qualities attributed to the soul in the last sūtra are attained).

COMMENTARY

The material condition is of constant inferiority, jealousy, and the search for greatness. Under this condition, the soul is naturally averse to the epitome of greatness—namely, the Supreme Lord. The soul wants to be just like the Lord, but instead of becoming great, he becomes the servant of the material body and the mind. When instead he realizes his true nature of happiness, knowledge, and eternal activity, he becomes devoted to the Supreme Lord who has the same nature, although much greater than the soul's. The very nature of inner happiness is that there is no inferiority, and under a joyful condition, the soul appreciates the greatness that is much greater than Him. The Lord is also eternally joyful and compassionate, and the soul enjoys the Lord's association. This association is not one of taking without giving. It is rather one of love and devotion in which one gives without an expectation of a return because there is no fear of running out of the infinite capacity of giving that lies within. Thus, both the Lord and the soul are happily devoted to each other, and give each other selflessly. In fact, they enjoy the act of pleasing each other continuously.

The earlier sūtras spoke about the process of detachment, destruction of material impressions and desires, and how they lead to the realization of the true nature of the self. And this sūtra states that the same result is attained by devotion to the Lord. This is contrary to the contentions of the impersonalist who says that any devotion involves qualities, and, by practicing these qualities, one cannot become free of qualities. After noting in the previous sūtra that the soul itself has qualities of softness and moderation, this sūtra goes a step further and says that the same qualities are obtained by devotion to the Lord. Therefore, the devotees of the Lord are also liberated souls, although they have attained this position through devotion rather than the process of hearing about the futility of material life, and the four steps of argument, thought, enjoyment, and egotism. The Vedic system acknowledges many paths to the same destination of spiritual perfection because different people are inclined differently. Their bodily and mental proclivities make some paths easier than others.

Sūtra 1.24

क्लेशकर्मविपाकाशयैरपरामृष्टःपुरुषविशेष ईश्वरः

kleśakarmavipākāśayairaparāmṛṣṭaḥ puruṣaviśeṣa īśvaraḥ

kleśa—suffering; karmavipāka—the adverse results of previous actions; āśayair—the resting places of; aparāmṛṣṭaḥ—unaffected; puruṣaviśeṣa—the special soul; īśvaraḥ—the Lord.

TRANSLATION

The Lord is that special soul who is unaffected by the resting places of the adverse results of the previous actions and the (resulting) suffering.

COMMENTARY

The soul has to endeavor to discover his true nature, but the Lord has no need for such a project. He is eternally liberated from the conditions of material entanglement. The previous sūtra stated that the soul is devoted to the Lord, and this sūtra explains why that is the case. The soul can be fallen, and then liberated. But the Lord is never fallen; He is ever liberated. This is because He never acts out of jealousy, malice, lust, greed, or selfishness. Hence, His actions are ever free from the adverse consequences of materialistic actions. The soul can forget his identity and his true nature, but the Lord is ever cognizant of His true nature. The soul can identify with a material body and mind—which are not the true self—but the Lord never commits such a folly. Thus, in various ways we can know how the Lord is not just different, but also superior to us. If this superiority is realized, then the soul is naturally devoted to the Lord.

Sūtra 1.25

तत्र निरतिशयं सर्वज्ञवीजम्

tatra niratiśayaṁ sarvajñavījam

tatra—there; niratiśayam—unsurpassable; sarvajña—omniscience; vījam—the seed.

TRANSLATION

In the Lord there is the seed for unsurpassable omniscience.

COMMENTARY

When the soul is liberated, then it can potentially know anything, but even then, it never knows everything. In that sense, the Lord is all-knowing, but the soul is not. Nevertheless, even when the Lord can know everything, He may focus His consciousness on what He wants to know. Thus, in the previous sūtra, it was stated that the Lord is not touched by the places of misery. We might ask: How can the Lord be called all-knowing, and yet not be aware of misery? And the answer is that the Lord chooses where to direct His awareness. So, His capacity for omniscience doesn't mean that He is constantly suffering the miseries being suffered by others. There is a difference between knowing pain, and being in pain. This difference is attained when the consciousness stops identifying with the pain, and observes the pain—as if someone else was in pain. Thus, the Lord has the power of omniscience, but that power may lie unutilized. Hence it is called a 'seed', which exists in a potential form, but may not fructify. Even though the Lord can become aware of the miseries of the world, He chooses not to be aware of them—if He so wants. As a result, He is untouched by these problems. But if He wants, He can also become aware of the material reality. Hence in the śrutī, it is said that the Lord has His 'back' toward the material energy. It is not that He cannot turn toward it; He chooses to remain unaware. The soul can also acquire this nature of the Lord, where even if adverse conditions exist, the soul can focus its consciousness on the spiritual endeavors.

Sūtra 1.26

पूर्वेषामपि गुरुःकालेनानवच्छेदात्

pūrveṣāmapi guruḥ kālenānavacchedāt

pūrveṣāmapi—even the previous; guruḥ—the spiritual masters; kālena—by time; anavacchedāt—due to not being covered or hidden.

TRANSLATION

(The Lord is the spiritual master of) even the previous spiritual masters, due to not being covered or hidden by time.

COMMENTARY

Spiritual knowledge is often lost due to the effect of time, despite the best efforts of enlightened teachers. This generally happens due to the predominance of atheistic people, who stop the saintly people from conducting their spiritual practices, and teaching the spiritual knowledge to others. It also happens when true understanding of yoga is lost and replaced by mundane ideas. At present, for example, yoga is equated to exercises, mixed with mundane psychology, and primarily used for keeping a healthy body and mind, instead of its true purpose, which is getting out of material entanglements. This is due to the effect of time. In short, the destruction of true knowledge is also an effect of time; similarly, the reestablishment of the truth is an effect of time. When the appropriate time arrives, true knowledge spreads; and when the appropriate time arrives, the truth is automatically hidden. In this age called Kali-yuga, all principles of truth, right, and good are compromised for short-term gains. People are unable to see anything beyond their bodily existence, and how this body is created, how it changes, and how the soul remains unchanged is ignored. Thus, true knowledge naturally appears and disappears by the effect of time.

However, this sūtra also notes that when this knowledge appears through a spiritual master, the Lord is always the source of that knowledge. This is particularly instructive for this age where many charlatan gurus claim to have attained perfection by their "meditation" without prior having a guru, who in turn had a guru, all the way to the Lord. The fake gurus in this age disregard the statements of the previous preceptors and invent their own philosophy and system of religion, and the foolish followers who have no knowledge of the spiritual tradition emanating from the Lord accept such cheaters as their teachers. By following a fake guru, their spiritual progress is also doomed. By the prevalence of such false gurus most common people are confused about the true path because each such false guru says something different from the other false gurus, which is at variance from the gurus of the past and the scriptures. The true guru is judged by his accordance to the preceding gurus and the scriptures, and ultimately based on the instruction of the Lord who originates the spiritual instruction. Hence, anyone who disregards devotion to the Lord, the previous spiritual masters, or the statements of the scriptures, must be immediately rejected as a cheater. It doesn't matter how many followers they have, how sensible their words appear to be, etc. When a person is disconnected from the spiritual tradition, the scriptures, and the Lord, he loses spiritual power. He might have some temporary material power, name, fame, prestige, wealth, etc. But those things do not lead a prospective disciple to spiritual progress.

Sūtra 1.27
तस्य वाचकःप्रणवः
tasya vācakaḥ praṇavaḥ

tasya—of that (Lord), vācakaḥ—name, speaker; praṇavaḥ—the sound om.

TRANSLATION
The name of that (Lord) is the sound "om".

COMMENTARY
The Lord has infinite names, and each name represents a certain quality of the Lord. The sound "om" represents the self-realized nature of the Lord. The sound "om", comprises three letters a, u, and m, which are the primordial representations of the three capacities of the soul, called, sat, chit, and ānanda. The Lord is the fullness of these three qualities, and in the monosyllable "om", these three qualities are merged. That merger of these three qualities represents self-awareness of the nature of the self— i.e., sat, chit, and ānanda. The term ānanda represents the knower who desires to know. Then, the term sat represents the consciousness which is directed toward the self. And as a result of that direction of consciousness to the self, the nature of the self is known as someone who can know. That knowing self, which uses its power to know, to know that it is capable of knowing its own true nature, is the meaning of the sound "om".

You might think that this is such a trivial proposition, but it is not. The caveat in this proposition is that I can know myself unassisted by anything else. In this world, we are trying to know ourselves through other people, relationships, things, acquisitions, achievements, and so on. We think we are rich if we acquire some wealth. We think we are knowledgeable if we acquire knowledge of other things. In this way, our self-realization is mediated via other things. The "om" state is the self-realization that is unmediated by other things.

All other letters of Sanskrit expand from the sound "om" and thereafter from these letters all kinds of texts—including the Vedic texts—are produced. The basic principle of this expansion is that once the self-aware state called sat-chit-ānanda is understood, then the expansion of the sound is merely the elaboration of the nature of the self. In short, the world is produced by expressing the self into many things. Thus, knowledge, beauty, power, wealth, fame, etc. are manifest as things that were originally part of the self, and are not separated. Therefore, the self-realized state is the ground from which everything else springs, in the process of becoming aware of the detailed meaning of sat, chit, and ānanda. That detailing of these three qualities produces all variety and the manifest reality is nothing other than the ways in which a conscious person can know itself. When the sound "om" divides into many parts, and the connection to the original sound "om" is ignored, then a false understanding of the divided sounds is produced; in that false understanding, there are many separated and individual qualities, disconnected from the source of self-realization. Then we think that language is arbitrary human invention, rather than something that originates in self-awareness, in the goal to know oneself, and creates the variety from the self in the attempt to expand and understand one's own nature.

All the Vedic mantras use the sound "om", which is also called praṇava, as the first sound, following which other qualities are described. For instance, in the mantra "om namo bhagavate vāsudevāya" the sound "om" comes first, which indicates that the self-realized soul (represented by "om") offers obeisance to Lord Vāsudeva. The basic meaning of "om" is self-realized state, and everything springs from that state. These mantras are therefore not mundane sounds, because their first sound is "om" and everything else that follows is the byproduct or manifestation from the self-realized state. By repeating these sounds, we enter the realization of an aspect of the self-realized state. For instance, if we chant "om namo bhagavate vāsudevāya", then we enter that state of self-realization ("om") in which we will offer obeisance to Vāsudeva. This mantra thus represents the self-realization that the self is a part of Vāsudeva. Just like the hands and legs of the body serve the body, similarly, Vāsudeva is the whole, and the self-realized soul is His part and offers obeisance to Him. Thus, the self-realization is always in relation to the Supreme Personality.

This sūtra can also be translated as "The spiritual master of the previous spiritual masters is the sound om". Thereby, the yoga philosophy also becomes the emanation of the sound "om", which means that this philosophy is not the product of a mundane mind; it is the byproduct of the self-realized state. Similarly, the Lord is called by the sound "om" and from His self-realization about His nature, all the knowledge about the self-realization manifests. This sound is called śabda-brahman, which is the sound representation of Brahman. We can ask: What is Brahman? It is a state of self-realization in which the soul is absorbed in the understanding of the nature of the self, which has three aspects—sat, chit, and ānanda. The śabda-brahman is the sound representation of that knowledge of the self; it is the word by which this knowledge is represented. Thus, by chanting "om" we can enter the self-realized state called Brahman. However, if "om" alone is chanted, then the self-realization is incomplete, because the self is known, but the purpose of the self's existence is not known. If instead "om namo bhagavate vāsudevāya" is chanted, then the self is known, and it is understood that the purpose of the self is serving the Lord Vāsudeva. This kind of self-realization is complete as it includes the self and its innate purpose. Therefore, any self-realization that is devoid of the realization of the Lord is devoid of the complete and true understanding of the meaning of "om". This sūtra states that the Lord is called by the name "om", and the previous sūtra stated that the Lord is the origin of all knowledge of the spiritual masters. Therefore, the sound "om" has two meanings. First, it refers to the Lord's knowledge of Himself. Second, it refers to the self-realized state in general. The soul's self-realized state is based on the self-realized state of the Lord.

The Brahman is not a *thing*, but a *state*. The Supreme Lord originally exists in this state, and then He is called Param-Brahman. From the Param-Brahman state everything else is expanded, including the soul. Once these things are expanded, they have the power to know the self, or even to ignore the nature of the self. Thus, the soul can draw its consciousness away from the self and become ignorant of the self. It can also draw the consciousness inward and realize that there is a self to be known independent of the mediated methods of knowing. Finally, the self can draw the consciousness further inward and seek its purpose of existence. That deepest level of self-understanding is also the Lord's understanding because the purpose of self-existence is the Lord. Since in the Brahman state the self is known, but the purpose of its existence is not known, therefore, the Brahman is an inactive state. For instance, we can know that we are capable of speech, but we may not speak, because the purpose to be fulfilled by that speech is unknown. When that purpose is also realized, then the soul may chant the mantra "om namo bhagavate vāsudevāya" even in the self-realized state, indicating that the purpose of his existence is Lord Vāsudeva.

Therefore, when the Brahman state is identified with the soul's own state, then it is incomplete. However, when that state is identified with the Lord's self-aware nature, then it is complete. All expansions of that state produce other sounds, and the Vedic scriptures are therefore said to be "spoken" by the Lord, because they are emanations from His self-realized state. Similarly, those who have perfected their understanding of the self—in relationship to the Lord—can also speak the scriptures, and whatever they speak becomes a scripture, because scripture is nothing but the emanation of a self-realized state. As a result, the Vedic scriptures include not just those things spoken by the Lord, but also those things that are spoken by other self-realized souls. There is no fundamental difference between the speech that emerges from self-realization of the soul and the self-realization of the Lord. Therefore, even if one says that the Yoga Sūtras were composed by Sage Pātañjali, rather than spoken by the Lord, there is no fundamental difference if the speaker is in the self-realized state. They don't just speak the truth; rather, whatever they speak is the truth.

In the Brahman state there is no speech, other than "om", and this is the imperfection in the Brahman state because the eternal existence of the self is recognized but the fact that this existence is meaningless is not recognized. This is clarified when we understand that the "om" refers to the Lord's self-realized state and not our state. Since the Lord is never forgetful about His nature, therefore, He is always self-realized and the name "om" refers to Him. Since He is the origin of everything, therefore, true self-realization is understanding our relationship to the Lord. If our self-realization was the complete and perfect state, then the various Vedic mantras and the Vedic texts would not exist. These texts and mantras are spoken by those who have transcended the Brahman state and realized not just their eternal existence, but also the eternal purpose of that existence. When they speak, that speech is itself considered the perfect truth. The Yoga philosophy is one such speech: It is also the perfect truth. We can say that it was spoken by the Lord, that it was composed by Sage Pātañjali, or that it is an emanation of the sound "om". All these are equivalent statements.

Sūtra 1.28
तज्जपस्तदर्थभावनम्
tajjapastadarthabhāvanam

tat—that; japas—chant; tadartha—that meaning (i.e., "om"); bhāvanam—meditation with great devotion.

TRANSLATION
Chant that, meditate with great devotion on that meaning (i.e., "om").

COMMENTARY
An earlier sūtra described that the perfected soul is devoted to the Lord. Then the last sūtra stated that the Lord is called by the sound "om". Now, this sūtra prescribes the chanting of the Lord's name with great devotion. This chanting is both the process of meditation on the Lord, and the state of the perfected soul after their liberation from the material entanglement. The devotion to the Lord is the eternal nature of the soul. So, the chanting of the names of the Lord is not merely for liberation; it continues even after liberation.

Sūtra 1.29
ततःपरत्यक्चेतनाधगिमोऽप्यन्तरायाभावश्च
tataḥ pratyakcetanādhigamo'pyantarāyābhāvaśca

tataḥ—from that (chanting); pratyakcetana—the individual consciousness; adhigamaḥ—knowledge; api—even; antarāya—separation; abhāvaḥ—absence.

TRANSLATION
From that (chanting), the individual consciousness even gets the knowledge (of the Lord) and even (the feeling of) separation and absence.

COMMENTARY

The chanting of the names of the Lord is just like calling a person lovingly. We call a person when we miss them, or when we want to be close to them. In the same way, when a devotee calls the Lord by His name, he develops the feeling of separation, and by that separation, he gets the vision of the Lord. Chanting the names of the Lord is thus the prescribed method for meditation in this age, because it establishes the loving devotion to the Lord, and by that devotion all materialistic tendencies are automatically destroyed. Since the loving devotion to the Lord exists even in the liberated condition, therefore, the chanting of the names of the Lord is both the goal as well as the means by which the goal is attained. This process simplifies the spiritual practice noticeably.

Readers might have noticed that thus far the text has not mentioned anything about a yogic posture, doing breathing exercises, or other such things, which are commonly identified by the term 'yoga'. All that has been stated thus far is that one must control the tendencies of the chitta, by which one realizes the true nature of the self, which is eternally happy and devoted to the Lord. Thus, those who focus exclusively on breath control or exercises misrepresent the nature of yoga, contrary to the prescriptions of the Yoga Sūtra itself.

Sūtra 1.30

व्याधिस्त्यानसंशयप्रमादालस्याविरतिभ्रान्तिदर्शनालब्ध
भूमिकत्वानवस्थितत्वानि चित्तविक्षेपास्तेऽन्तरायाः

**vyādhistyānasaṁśayapramādālasyāviratibhrāntidarśanālabdha
bhūmikatvānavasthitatvāni cittavikṣepāste'ntarāyāḥ**

vyādhi—sickness; styāna—stupidity; saṁśaya—doubt; pramāda—negligence; ālasya—laziness; avirati—attachment; bhrānti-darśana—watching illusory things; ālabdha—desires for that which has not been obtained; bhūmikatva—pride in the position; anavasthitatvāni—unsteadiness, and such; chitta—the chitta; vikṣepāste—being throwing into; antarāyāḥ—hindrances.

TRANSLATION

Sickness, stupidity, doubt, negligence, laziness, attachment, watching illusory things, desires for that which is not obtained, pride in the position, unsteadiness, and such, throw the chitta into the hindrances (in the yoga practice).

COMMENTARY

After noting the spiritually enlightened state in which the soul is devoted to the Lord, many conditions are described by which the soul abandons the process of yoga. These can be viewed as (1) things to be renounced by those who are beginning the process, (2) hindrances on the path of practitioners, (3) warnings to those who might consider themselves perfect, and (4) ways by which other people can judge whether a person is truly spiritually advanced, or whether he is merely pretending to be in that state. The first such state is sickness of the body. If the body is sick, it affects the mind and that ultimately compels a person to abandon the process of yoga, or creates hurdles in it.

The rest of the hurdles are attributable to the mind. For instance, doing stupid things, doubting that the process of yoga can lead one to perfection, laziness in following the rules and regulations, attachments to mundane things, watching illusory things like movies or reading newspapers or listening to mundane songs, feeling very proud of one's current or past achievements, or hankering for that which has yet not been achieved, or simply wavering in one's practices for no good reason, are all pitfalls in the path to the perfection of yoga.

Sūtra 1.31

दुःखदौर्मनस्याङ्गमेजयत्वश्वासप्रश्वासा विक्षेपसहभुवः

duḥkhadaurmanasyāṅgamejayatvaśvāsapraśvāsā
vikṣepasahabhuvaḥ

duḥkha—unhappiness; daurmanasya—bad thoughts; aṅgam—the body parts; ejayatva—shaking or agitation; śvāsapraśvāsa—heavy breathing; vikṣepa—fall; sahabhuvaḥ—arise with.

TRANSLATION

Unhappiness, bad thoughts, the agitation of the body parts, heavy breathing arise with a fallen state (caused by the conditions of the previous sūtra).

COMMENTARY

This sūtra describes further consequences of the modifications of the chitta. The first such consequence is unhappiness. Why should unhappiness arise? The answer is that the chitta gives rise to a modification, and that modification interacts with the ego, and creates a sense of inadequacy. For example, if the thought of tasty food arises in the chitta, then it interacts with the ego, and it gives rise to the desire for tasty food. This desire is unhappiness, because all desires represent what we are missing. A desire is like a hole or a socket which has to be filled by some content or form, and the object of that desire is that form. Happiness is gained when the content or form fills the hole. But for it to fill the hole, the hole must exist. And this hole constitutes unhappiness.

When this unhappiness interacts with the intellect and the mind, bad thoughts arise. For example, we may not have access to tasty food, or it may be hard work to cook that tasty food, or that tasty food may be very expensive. Then we go through a convoluted process of how to acquire that tasty food with the least amount of effort, and often this means that we are cutting corners, neglecting the moral principles, being disturbed by the inability to figure out how to get this pleasure, and so on. Similarly, when the thought of tasty food arises in the chitta, by the interaction with the senses, the mouth starts watering. Now, it is not just the ego which is feeling inadequate; it is also the senses which start desiring the tasty food. As this desire intensifies, the body is set into motion where it cooks tasty food, travels to a restaurant to eat tasty food, or finds other ways to steal or coerce others into giving us tasty food. And with the movement of the body, the breathing becomes heavy, as we are no longer peaceful and restful. Thus, a progressive conversion of a primitive wave into a feeling of inadequacy, to crooked methods at fulfilling desires, to bodily agitation is noted. In this way, the modifications of the chitta control the bodily actions.

Sūtra 1.32

तत्परतषिधार्थमेकतत्त्वाभ्यासः

tatpratiṣedhārthamekatattvābhyāsaḥ

tatpratiṣedha—the cessation of these (modifications); artham—the purpose of; ekatattva—the one principle; abhyāsaḥ—the practice.

TRANSLATION

The practice of focusing on one principle is for the purpose of the cessation of these (modifications).

COMMENTARY

When our consciousness is focused on the Lord, it is automatically defocused from the material body and the mind. The material bodies and minds are many and diverse. The souls are also many and diverse. So, what can be that "one principle"? It is certainly the Supreme Lord. Thus, after stating that the purpose of yoga is the cessation of chitta's modifications, then stating that the liberated soul is devoted to the Lord, then describing how such liberated devotees call the Lord's name, this sūtra states that this progressive process—from the silencing of the chitta, to discovery of the self, to the devotion to the Lord—can be substituted by pursuing the path of devotion from the outset. That is called "focusing on the one principle", rather than separately focusing on silencing the chitta, the nature of the self, and then the nature of the Lord. By devotion to the Lord, the effects of chitta silencing, and the realization of the soul different from the body, and attainment of happiness, are all obtained.

Sūtra 1.33

मैत्रीकरुणामुदितोपेक्षाणां सुखदुःखपुण्यापुण्यवषियाणां
भावनातश्चतितपरसादनम्

maitrīkaruṇāmuditopekṣāṇāṁ
sukhaduḥkhapuṇyāpuṇyaviṣayāṇāṁ bhāvanātaścittaprasādanam

maitrī—friendship; karuṇā—compassion; mudita—sexual pleasure; upekṣāṇām—ignoring; sukha-duḥkha-puṇya-apuṇya-viṣayāṇām —the subjects of happiness, distress, good and bad deeds; bhāvanātaḥ— the culmination of the devotional feeling; ca—also; citta—the chitta; prasādanam—gifts.

TRANSLATION

The ignoring of friendship, compassion (e.g., toward children and servants), sexual pleasure, the subjects of happiness, distress, good and bad deeds, are also the gifts of the chitta as the culmination of the devotional feeling.

COMMENTARY

The mundane life involves the enjoyment of several kinds of emotions. These include the sexual or romantic love, the feeling of affection toward children, the compassion toward those who are subordinates, and the feeling of camaraderie toward the friends. When one progresses somewhat from this mundane life, one starts thinking about the nature of right and wrong actions, and how they lead to happiness and distress. Most religious thinking focuses upon moralistic thinking where the central goal of life is to be liberated from the many kinds of suffering, and be situated in happiness. Similarly, most of religious thinking is focused on getting out of the entanglements of social life, such as friends, wife, children, and employment. This sūtra makes a stunning statement that all of these goals are easily achieved by devotion to the Lord. In short, whether you are trying to become detached from materialistic life, or you are pondering the nature of good and bad deeds, or you are considering what constitutes the best kind of happiness, you don't require varieties of theories, doctrines, practices, or processes. The devotion to the Lord achieves everything. It frees a person from suffering, and places them in the perfect happiness.

Sūtra 1.34
प्रच्छर्दनविधारणाभ्यां वा प्राणस्य
pracchardanavidhāraṇābhyāṁ vā prāṇasya

pracchardana—exhalation; vidhāraṇābhyām—retention; abhyam—the two; vā—moving or activity; prāṇasya—are the properties of prāṇa.

TRANSLATION

The two activities of exhalation and retention are the properties of prāṇa.

COMMENTARY

The prāṇa is actually five-fold, which includes prāṇa (ingestion), apāna (excretion), udāna (expression), vyāna (circulation), and samāna (digestion). In these five types of prāṇa, the process of expression and excretion are included in the 'exhalation' process. For example, when we speak, then we are exhaling through the mouth. Similarly, when we exhale through the nose, the process is called apāna. Thus, the yogic practice of the control of prāṇa includes the exhalation through the mouth as well as through the nose, and while they are just called 'exhalation' they represent the processes of udāna and apāna. The process of retention, similarly, includes the activities of vyāna and samāna. When the breath is held inward, then a pressure is created, and that pressure can be felt either in the upper part of the body (we can equate this with lungs) or in the lower part of the body (we can equate this with the stomach). The breath held in the stomach constitutes samāna and that held in the lung constitutes the vyāna. Thus, the processes of vyāna and samāna are combined and summarized in the activity of retention. Finally, there is the process of inhalation, which is called prāṇa in this sūtra as the power to establish a connection between two things. All other processes are varied manifestations of the prāṇa alone.

To understand this description, we must think of prāṇa as the power to make and break connections. When a new connection is established which previously did not exist, the process is called prāṇa. By this process, the food is ingested, the breath is taken in, the senses grasp the external objects, etc. Once they are ingested within, then they are transported within the body to the right place. For example, the food is moved into the stomach, the sounds are sent into the brain, the breath is moved into the lungs. This is called the process of vyāna. Once they have reached their intended destination, then they are broken down into units or pieces that can be absorbed. For example, the sounds are broken down into syllables and words by which they are cognized. The food is broken down into assimilable units. And the air that we breath in is broken down to the assimilable and non-assimilable parts. This process is called samāna. Then, some undigested food, inassimilable air, or unprocessed sounds are discarded. This process is called apāna. Then, whatever has been absorbed is transformed into an expression, such as speech, bodily activity, or work. This transformation of the prāṇa energy into other forms is also called udāna or expression.

Ultimately, all of these processes are simply the variations of making and breaking connections. But since they produce different outcomes, therefore, they are called by different ways. Thus, in one sense, there is only one power of making and breaking connections, which is called prāṇa. But we can also call this power by five different names if we divide it into five actions of ingestion, digestion, circulation, assimilation, and excretion. Finally, we can also present this as a three-fold process of ingestion, retention, and exhalation, with the latter two being the summarized divisions of two other processes. These varied descriptions do not seem inconsistent if we understand the nature of prāṇa.

Sūtra 1.35
वषियवती वा प्रवृत्तरिुत्पन्ना मनसःस्थतिनिबिन्धिनी
viṣayavatī vā pravṛttirutpannā manasaḥ sthitinibandhinī

viṣayavatī—relating to objects; vā—moving; pravṛttir-utpannā—produced by tendencies; manasaḥ—the mind; sthiti—position; nibandhinī—connected to.

TRANSLATION

Produced by the material tendencies, moving to relate to material objects, the mind's position is that of being connected to (the material world).

COMMENTARY

The mind is called the sixth sense in Vedic philosophy and is distinguished from the five senses of hearing, touching, seeing, tasting, and smelling. By the five senses we can obtain percepts and by the mind we obtain meanings. For example, as you read this book, the eyes are gathering the shapes and sizes of squiggles, and the mind is understanding the meaning of the words. To perceive these meanings, the mind must cognize a few different things. For example, the mind must divide the sounds into phonemes and words; this sometimes seems easy in English as the words are separated by spaces, but even then, the words themselves are comprised of phonemes, and the mind classifies the sounds into distinct sound-units. Then, the mind decodes the grammatical structure of sentences—e.g., which adjective is attached to which noun. It must understand the context in which things are spoken. And then, it must discern the intention of the speaker. In all such ways, the mind is outward-bound. It seeks to understand the nature of reality by interpreting the sense percepts.

The seeking of the mind is not merely dependent on what is 'out there' but also by its own conditioning. For example, we can distinguish between words in a text only because we are familiar with a particular language vocabulary. We can understand the grammatical structure, because we have learned it prior. And we can understand the speaker's intentions only if we have a similar type of intention. Thus, the mind is not a 'blank slate'. It is rather an instrument that seeks certain ideas and neglects others. It is an instrument with predefined molds into which only certain things fit, while the other things are discarded.

In these ways, the mind is considered the outbound instrument of perception, just like the other five senses. This is important because unless these tendencies at outward bound movement are curbed, we cannot understand the nature of the self. Unless we can see how we are different from this mind, we cannot obtain control over the mind. And without this control, there can be no spiritual life. Thus, it is important to know how the mind can detract us from the spiritual path, and be cautious of its tendencies, before we even use it.

Sūtra 1.36
वशिोका वा ज्योतष्मिती
viśokā vā jyotiṣmatī

viśokā—unhappiness; vā—moving; jyotiṣmatī—toward enlightenment.

TRANSLATION

Move the mind from unhappiness toward enlightenment.

COMMENTARY

After noting that the mind is outward bound, and dictated by materialistic tendencies, this sūtra exhorts the reader to move the mind toward enlightenment. How can this be achieved, if the mind is always outward bound? And the answer is that even in the external world, there are sources of true knowledge, such as books, mantras, spiritual practices, and the deities of the Lord. By focusing the mind on these external things, we can take it toward enlightenment. So, the outward-bound nature of the mind is a problem if the objects with which the mind engages are materialistic. And the same outward-bound nature of the mind is the source of spiritual enlightenment if it is engaged properly. We can see how this idea is different from the cessation of the modifications of the chitta: We were earlier treating the mind, and its modifications, as the enemy of spiritual realization. We are now treating the same mind as the friend of spiritual progress. And this is achieved if we changed the *focus* of the mind. The mind is by itself hence neither the enemy nor the friend. The mind is just an instrument, that can be used either for elevation or the degradation of the soul.

Sūtra 1.37
वीतरागवषियं वा चतितम्
vītarāgaviṣayaṁ vā cittam

vītarāga—become detached; viṣayam—the material objects; vā—extricating or removing; chittam—the chitta.

TRANSLATION

Become detached from the material objects by removing the chitta.

COMMENTARY

As we have discussed earlier, the chitta is our history which imbues us with the notions of ideality, or what is perfection. When the chitta interacts with the mind, then the meanings obtained from the world are treated as the ideal meanings. For example, someone can look at pictures of a happy family and think: "This is the ideal family life". A person reading a book on romantic poetry can think: "This is the ideal version of love life". Or, a materialistic person can look at a rich and handsome man, and think: "This is the ideal example of a man". Thus, the mind gathers knowledge of the world, and the chitta judges these things to be ideal. When they are judged to be ideal, the consciousness is drawn toward them, and that is called the mind's attraction toward the material objects. This sūtra exhorts the reader to become detached from the worldly objects. That can happen only if we transform our notion of perfection and ideality, because then when we see the things in the world, we will not find them ideal.

This doesn't mean that we stop looking at the world. It just means that we look at it, and say: "This is not ideality or perfection". It has got so many faults, and whatever seems perfect is also illusory. The picture of a happy family is just a picture; it doesn't necessarily mean that there is actually a happy family. The beauty of love portrayed in romantic poetry is just poetry; people don't find such poetic romantic love in the real world. And this rich and handsome man may look attractive on the outside, but if we look closer, we will find the same traits of greed, jealousy, anger, and hatefulness as we can see in poor men.

Sūtra 1.38

स्वप्ननिद्राज्ञानालम्बनं वा
svapnanidrājñānālambanaṁ vā

svapna—dream; nidrā—deep sleep; jñāna—knowledge; ālambanam—support; vā—not.

TRANSLATION
Dreaming and sleeping are not the support systems for knowledge.

COMMENTARY
The Vedic description of experience identifies four tiers. These are called waking, dreaming, deep sleep, and transcendent. In some ways, the dreaming and deep sleep experiences are considered superior to the waking state because they reveal more subtle levels of reality. However, dreaming and deep sleep are also considered to be dominated by the mode of tamo-guna. While the Lord and the spiritual master can sometimes appear in a dream to instruct an aspiring devotee, these instructions can as well be passed by the Paramātma in the heart while awake. It is only when we disregard these waking inspirations that the Lord or the spiritual master appear in a dream to provide an instruction. For all practical reasons, however, the dreaming and deep sleep states are not considered suitable means for imparting spiritual education. The dreaming state also includes reckless speculation and imagination; these are like dreaming even during waking. And knowledge acquired via speculative means is also not considered suitable for spiritual advancement. Only the knowledge that automatically springs in the heart, without preceding speculative thoughts, can be considered the direct inspiration from the Lord, and the Lord's guidance.

Sūtra 1.39
यथाभिमतध्यानाद्वा
yathābhimatadhyānādvā

yathā-abhimata—just as one thinks; dhyānāt—from meditation; vā—or.

TRANSLATION

Alternatively, just as one thinks, from meditation the same thing is known.

COMMENTARY

Many people claim that they found the truth by meditation, where by meditation they simply mean sitting in a posture and concentrating their mind. If this were indeed true, then every meditator who has a wandering mind could claim to have seen some "truth" since their mind was anyway wandering.

The previous sūtra refuted that dreaming and deep sleep are methods for real knowledge. This sūtra states that even so-called waking meditation is not a method of knowledge. It only reveals what we have already been thinking. For example, if we have two beliefs, one that is stronger and the other that is weaker, during meditation the weaker belief would be further weakened, and the stronger belief will stand strong. Thus, because the weaker belief is shut down, therefore, this meditation will only reveal what was already the stronger belief. This is not considered a method of knowledge because it can also confirm false beliefs. This process of meditation is often used by people to gain greater self-confidence. For instance, you might want to do something, and you may be theoretically convinced that it is the right thing to do, but you also might have doubts. If you concentrate the mind, your prior conviction will become stronger, and the doubts or disbeliefs will become weaker. Hence, by meditation you will become even more convinced of your prior convictions. This is good if the prior convictions were indeed true. But it can be very bad if the prior convictions were false. Thus, it is important to acquire the correct belief through the spiritual master, the information from the scripture, or the true authorities, and meditate on that. Similarly, we can meditate on the names of the Lord. Arbitrary meditation only reinforces what we were already convinced of.

Meditation doesn't mean concentrating our attention on the tip of the nose, into the middle of the eyebrows, at the top of the head, at the center of our belly, into the region of the heart, and so on. These are not valid objects of meditation. While these types of meditations will be described later in this text, they are meant for obtaining different kinds of material knowledge, not spiritual advancement. The valid objects of meditation are the names and forms of the Lord, or the knowledge of the Absolute Truth given in the scriptures. Nevertheless, as many people whimsically invent other objects of meditation, therefore, it is important to clarify that when we perform such kinds of meditations, then the weaker beliefs are dimmed, and the stronger beliefs become stronger. And the net result of such meditation is that one acquires a stronger conviction, but that could well be the conviction in something that is simply not true.

Sūtra 1.40

परमाणुपरममहत्त्वान्तोऽस्य वशीकारः

paramāṇuparamamahattvānto'sya vaśīkāraḥ

paramāṇu—the atoms; paramama—the smallest; hattva—killed; antah—the end or limit; asya—of this; vaśīkāraḥ—control is obtained.

TRANSLATION

When the limit of the destruction of the smallest atoms of this (chitta) is reached, then control (over the chitta) is obtained.

COMMENTARY

The Vedic idea of atomism is quite different from the atomism in modern science. To understand this atomism, we must prior understand that everything in this world is constructed out of ideas, and there are big ideas and small ideas. The big idea is necessarily a more abstract idea, and the small idea is necessarily a more detailed idea. When we start purifying the chitta, we always attack the big ideas. An example of a big false idea is materialism; for instance, in the present condition we might think that there is no soul, and we are merely the body. An attack on materialism would therefore try to establish the existence of the soul. Now, many people might accept the proofs of the soul apart from the body. But that acceptance doesn't mean that they are free of materialism. It may well be a theoretical acknowledgment that the body alone is not sufficient to explain how life emerged, why we desire a purposeful life, why we are inclined to moral behavior, and so on. And yet, despite this acknowledgement, for all practical purposes, a person might continue doing the same materialistic activities as the others who don't accept the soul's existence. For instance, even a person who accepts the soul's existence may still consider earning wealth, taking care of their family, or social relationships their top priority, while the needs of the soul are neglected. So, such a person is not truly out of materialism.

To be completely free of materialism, we have to cut out the last vestige of the identification with the body. The smallest symptom of materialism is the smallest 'atom' of materialism. Only when all vestiges have been removed, can we say that we are totally out of materialism. If even one symptom, symbolic representation, or vestige of material identity exists, then the abstract idea which is symbolized by this symptom also exists. This is hence the meaning of saying that until the smallest atoms are destroyed, we are not totally purified.

Sūtra 1.41

क्षीणवृत्तेरभिजातस्येव मणेर्ग्रहीतृग्रहणग्राह्येषु तत्स्थतदञ्जनता समापत्तिः

kṣīṇavṛtterabhijātasyeva maṇergrahītṛgrahaṇagrāhyeṣu tatsthatadañjanatā samāpattiḥ

kṣīṇa-vṛtteḥ—upon the weaking of the tendencies; abhijātasya—is born; eva—certainly; maṇeḥ—gem; grahītṛ—one who accepts; grahaṇa—the activity of accepting; grāhyeṣu—that which is accepted; tatstha—there is situated; tad-añjanatā—the ignorance of that (soul); samāpattiḥ—reaches the end.

TRANSLATION

Upon the weakening of the material tendencies is certainly born the gem (of the self). One who accepts, the activity of accepting, and the accepted object, are all situated in there (the self); the ignorance of that soul reaches an end.

COMMENTARY

Every form of knowledge or experience is constituted of three things—the knower, the known, and the process of knowing. In matter, however, these three things are always separated. That is, the body that knows is different from the body that is known, which is different from the process by which it is known. As long as there is material conditioning, we always think that the knower, the known, and the knowing are three separate things. However, when materialism begins to subside, then we realize that the knower, the known, and the knowing can be the same thing—i.e., the soul. These three aspects become identical when they pertain to the soul's self-awareness. So, cessation of materialism is identical to saying that there is a thing which is simultaneously the knower, the known, and the knowing, and that thing is the self or the soul.

Sūtra 1.42

शब्दार्थज्ञानवकिल्पैःसङ्कीर्णा सवितर्का समापत्तिः
śabdārthajñānavikalpaiḥ saṅkīrṇā savitarkā samāpattiḥ

śabdārtha—word and meaning; jñāna—the theories; vikalpaiḥ—alternatives; saṅkīrṇā—narrow; savitarkā—with the arguments; samāpattiḥ—end.

TRANSLATION

(With the realization of the soul), words and meanings, the theories and their narrow alternatives, come to an end along with hairsplitting arguments.

COMMENTARY

One who has practical realization can provide the simple descriptions of truth that others can understand. But when people who don't have such realization try to compete with a spiritually realized person, they create sophisticated vocabulary and definitions, propose complicated theories, and discuss their alternatives. This complicated philosophical jargon is ultimately not a substitute for true realization. It is mere sophistry that covers the ignorance of a pretentious person in the eyes of other ignorant people. The person who has true realization has no need for various complicated theories and philosophical jargon. He rather possesses the capacity to simplify everything into easy and simple ideas, which everyone understands. The person engaged in sophistry is generally stumped by this simplicity and claims that the truth cannot be so simple—after all he has been using such complicated jargon and is still unable to explain and understand it. But if such people follow the guidance of a self-realized person, then they can realize the truth. At that point, all the complicated theoretical jargon comes to an end, because the truth is all of the seemingly contradictory claims at once, and yet probably none of them individually.

Sūtra 1.43
स्मृतिपरिशुद्धौ स्वरूपशून्येवार्थमात्रनिरभासा निर्वितर्का
smṛtipariśuddhau svarūpaśūnyevārthamātranirbhāsā nirvitarkā

smṛti-pariśuddhau—upon the purification of memory; svarūpa—the soul's own form; śūnye—in the void; vā—going; arthamātra—just a goal; nirbhāsā—imaginary; nirvitarkā—that is without justification.

TRANSLATION

Upon the purification of memory, the soul's own form going into the void becomes just an imaginary goal that is without justification.

COMMENTARY

The previous sūtra stated that upon self-realization, the philosophical arguments come to an end. The philosophy of voidism now says: I told you so! There is no reality, no truth, and nothing to be achieved. If we just let go of all claims and counterclaims, then that state of complete emptiness is the truth.

This sūtra however talks about the 'purification of memory'. Memory holds our beliefs, or what we consider to be true. The philosophy of voidism says that our identity or what we call the 'self' is also a memory. For example, we have no memory of past lives, but we have some memories of this present life. Therefore, if all these memories were destroyed, then the person would be without an identity. And when there is no recollection (either of the self or of the world to which the self is connected by relations), then there is nothing to talk about. This sūtra rejects this understanding. The self is not merely memory. Even if all the memory is destroyed, only the current material identity will be destroyed, but the soul will not cease to exist. Yes, it can experience the void, but the experience of the void is still an experience, which requires an *experiencer*. Thus, the self—even when there is experience of a void—exists eternally. So, we have to purify our beliefs about who we really are, understand our identity, after removing the false identities. The cessation of material memories is not the end of the soul's identity because beyond that is the true knowledge of the self.

Sūtra 1.44
एतयैव सविचारा निर्विचारा च सूक्ष्मविषया व्याख्याता
etayaiva savicārā nirvicārā ca sūkṣmaviṣayā vyākhyātā

etayaiva—in this way certainly; savicārā—the good thought; nirvicārā—what should not be thought; ca—also; sūkṣmaviṣayā—subtle subjects; vyākhyātā—described as, or well known.

TRANSLATION
In this way certainly, the good thoughts and that which should not be thought are well known or described as subtle subjects.

COMMENTARY
The philosophy of voidism says that there is nothing to be thought of and emptying the mind is the goal of life. But this sūtra says that there is a difference between the acceptable and unacceptable thoughts. We cannot reject all thoughts. But the distinction between the accepted and rejected thoughts is very subtle. They are both thoughts, and therefore, thinking is itself not the problem. The problem is thinking false ideas, and we should endeavor to remove false thoughts alone. The true thoughts cannot be rejected just because we have earlier exclusively entertained false thoughts about what our identity is not.

Sūtra 1.45
सूक्ष्मविषयत्वं चालिङ्गपर्यवसानम्
sūkṣmaviṣayatvaṁ cāliṅgaparyavasānam

sūkṣmaviṣayatvaṁ—the subtle subjects; ca—also; aliṅga—the non-gendered; paryavasānam—at the end.

TRANSLATION

The subtle subjects also are at the end of a non-gendered reality.

COMMENTARY

Sāṅkhya philosophy identifies three kinds of bodies—sthūla, liṅga, and sūkṣma—or gross body, gendered body, and subtle body. The gendered body includes the senses, mind, intellect, ego, and morality, which means that male and female genders have different kinds of senses, mind (thoughts), intellect (beliefs), egos (goals), and morality (idealism). This gendered body, along with the gross body is created after birth from a subtle body which comprises the chitta, guna, and karma, under the influence of time. The chitta constitutes the unconscious impressions of the past, the guna are the unconscious likes, dislikes, and habits of enjoyment from the past, and the karma constitutes the unconscious consequences of the past actions. These three constitute a realm that is identified with the 'deep sleep' state of existence. The state of voidism pertains to this deep sleep state, where the consciousness of gender and gross body is lost, and hence can be called aliṅga or beyond the gendered state. However, entering this unconscious non-gendered state is not self-realization. The soul lies beyond these three kinds of bodies, and has the capacity to control them. Therefore, the state of voidism is not rejected as being false. But it is identified as a non-gendered, and yet, a material state, which is also called sūkṣma.

Sūtra 1.46
ता एव सवीजःसमाधिः
tā eva savījaḥ samādhiḥ

tā—that (deep sleep); eva—certainly; savījaḥ—with a seed; samādhiḥ—merged into the origin.

TRANSLATION

That (deep sleep) is certainly being merged into the origin with a seed.

COMMENTARY

Sāṅkhya philosophy describes how the soul is injected into the material energy called pradhāna which is the seed of all material creation.

The pradhāna is also called the unmanifest state, and we have previously discussed how the chitta manifests from pradhāna. The term pradhāna means the leader or the boss, and constitutes the ideas of lordship and leadership in this world. When the soul contacts the material reality, it thinks of a lordship by which it can become the boss or the superior personality in this world—and then act just like God. This preference for a particular kind of lordship is due to our past or history, but as new impressions are acquired, the idea of mastery keeps changing. Therefore, even as a person becomes some kind of master (facilitated by his past karma), his idea of mastery evolves. Hence, both due to the evolution of the idea of mastery, and due to loss of the previous mastery due to the finishing of karma, the soul can never truly become the master. And yet he tries hard.

The pradhāna is the objectified representation of the Lord's Śakti or power. This power is a potential energy which is activated by Śakti's will, under the guidance of the Lord's will. When the soul sees this potential energy, he thinks: Ah, now I can use this potential energy to become the master and boss. The soul doesn't realize that it is not *his* energy; it belongs to Śakti and always acts under Her control. But She allows the soul to play with the power according to the soul's karma. When the karma ends, the energy or power is withdrawn. Playing with the material energy is like playing with borrowed toys. We are playing due to the grace of the person who has let us play with those toys. But if the owner of the toy so desires, then he can take away the toy, and we would be just like children crying for the toy, and feeling deprived and cheated.

This pradhāna is the limit of the material deep sleep state. The fact is that prior to the creation, the soul is absorbed in self-consciousness— due to the absence of any other alternative—and when it is injected into pradhāna, then he slowly wakes up, which is a euphemism for consciousness being drawn outwardly into something that is different from the soul. Thus, from the prior state of forced self-consciousness, the other-consciousness develops as soon as there is an opportunity. Therefore, even if the soul again goes back into the pradhāna state, it is still not considered spiritual realization. Similarly, even if the soul returns to God's body at the end of the material creation, it is still not considered spiritual realization; it only appears to be spiritual due to absence of alternatives. The moment the alternative is presented, the soul falls into matter.

When the soul enters the void state, the seed of trying to become great still exists, although it is not manifest. This desire to be the boss or great is the root of the material existence. Thus, even when the soul is merged into the unconscious state of thoughtlessness, there is still a subtle but unmanifest idea of bossiness, which then manifests into the various attempts at trying to become a boss during dreams or waking states. Although devoid of the conscious experience, this is not considered the liberated state of the soul. It is rather the state where the soul has the seed of materialistic existence, but no experience. The implication is that the voidism is not a liberated state, but a material state. It can be likened to the deep sleep state in which there is no conscious experience.

Sūtra 1.47
नरि्वचिारवैशारद्येऽध्यात्मप्रसादः
nirvicāravaiśāradye'dhyātmaprasādaḥ

nirvicāra—without any thoughts; vaiśāradye—in proficiency; adhyātma—freedom from suffering of the body and mind; prasādaḥ—the benediction.

TRANSLATION
In the proficiency in thoughtlessness is the benediction of freedom from the suffering of the body and the mind.

COMMENTARY
Sāñkhya philosophy identifies three kinds of sufferings called ādidaivika (caused by the natural circumstances), ādibhautika (caused by other living entities), and ādiatmika (caused by one's own body and mind). This sūtra refers to this last type of suffering—including mental and physical illnesses—and says that if we become thoughtless, then we can be free from the mental and bodily suffering. It is not the mitigation of all suffering as one can still suffer in the other two ways—i.e., due to the misery caused by other living entities or due to the natural circumstances. Thus, for example, many people perform meditation to simply quieten the mind, pacify their breathing, strengthen their convictions, and rid the body of many pains and aches which arise due to fear, restlessness, and anxiety. This sūtra also states that by entering the thoughtless state, a person can mitigate the suffering of the body and the mind. However, this is

not perfect liberation because we are still in the material life and we can be forced to suffer due to other living entities or natural calamities. The true liberation is when we are out of material existence completely and the possibility of the recurrence of each of the three types of miseries noted above is completely eliminated. This is not to say that we may not aspire for freedom from the suffering of the body and the mind, but only to indicate that this process is insufficient. Thus, this sūtra identifies the benefits of the entry into thoughtlessness, and by contrast to the three types of suffering, notes why it is also inadequate. The true yogi is one who has completely destroyed each of three kinds of miseries.

Sūtra 1.48
ऋतम्भरा तत्र प्रज्ञा
ṛtambharā tatra prajñā

ṛtambharā—the knowledge of the truth; tatra—there; prajñā—the intellect.

TRANSLATION
The knowledge of the truth is there within the intellect.

COMMENTARY
One of the essential ideas in all Vedic philosophy is that falsity springs from the truth. What is falsity and what is truth? Truth is that which is obtained by the reconciliation of opposites, and falsity is that which is only one of these opposites. In the material world, these opposite ideas are very hard to reconcile, and they compete for attention and domination. In the spiritual world, these opposites are reconciled. Thus, the reconciled state of the opposites is truth, and the contradictory state of these opposites is the falsity. Once this idea is understood, then the primordial intelligence is defined as the embodiment of the truth in which the opposites are reconciled. This is also called 'pure' intelligence. However, under the material influence, its purity is lost, and the reconciliation of opposites turns into their contradiction. Then we think that only one of the two opposites can be true, and because each opposite is incomplete by itself, we enter a situation of imperfection and incompleteness. Over time, the intellect oscillates from one extreme to another, changing its beliefs, hoping that if one side of

the opposition doesn't work, then the other side must be perfect.

The reconciliation of the opposites can occur in two ways. First, we can reject both sides of the opposition, and say that *neither* of them is true. Second, we can accept both sides of the opposition and say that *both* of them are true. The state of voidism pertains to the 'neither' state and style of reconciling—all thoughts, propositions, theories, and doctrines are rejected as being false. The state of true intellect instead pertains to the 'both' state—all thoughts, propositions, theories, and doctrines are given a place within the complete truth. Thus, after rejecting the voidistic notion of there being no truth, this sūtra indicates how there is a truth, but it reconciles the opposites of this world. The voidistic state of 'neither' is thus rejected, but the state of 'both' is accepted.

This 'both' state is further identified as the waking state, not the deep sleep state. The buddhi, as we have discussed, has five states called correct and incorrect cognition, doubt, memory, and sleep. The sleep state is the forgetfulness of all knowledge, but the memory state is when everything is completely remembered. If this state is perfected, then one obtains the realization of the nature of the truth. If the memory is imperfect, then many thoughts spring in the mind, and the intellect tries to judge them as true or false, and a doubt is created, because the truth is not seen. Under these doubts, some memory is forgotten, and other memory is remembered. The philosophy of voidism says that we should clear all thoughts, and make our mind totally free of opinions, and judgments. That is indeed described to the be state of deep sleep of the intellect in Sāṅkhya philosophy. However, better than this is state is the memory state in which everything is remembered perfectly, and devoid of all the doubts. These doubts are resolved when all the contradictory positions are at once true. This doesn't mean that they are *equally* true. There is instead a hierarchy between superior and inferior truths, and due to this hierarchy, each contradictory idea is given a place in the pantheon of ideas. So, being true at once, doesn't mean equally true. Hence there is a distinction between Absolute and Relative truths. Both are truths, but the former is also superior to the latter type of truth.

Sūtra 1.49
श्रुतानुमानप्रज्ञाभ्यामन्यविषया विशेषार्थत्वात्

śrutānumānaprajñābhyāmanyaviṣayā viśeṣārthatvāt

śrutā—heard; anumāna—inference; prajñābhyām—by the intellect; anyaviṣayā—the other subjects; viśeṣārthatvāt—from the meaning of qualities.

TRANSLATION

That which is inferred by the intellect based upon that which was previous heard about the other subjects, is from the meaning of the qualities.

COMMENTARY

The perfect state of memory is that one doesn't forget the nature of the self, and hence doesn't identify himself with the body or the mind. Instead, the nature of the self is kept at the center of everything, and all other things are inferred based on that understanding. For example, the intellect no longer thinks that our consciousness could be produced due to matter. Rather, matter has the properties of cognizability by consciousness. So, whatever exists in matter also exists in consciousness, in the sense that everything that we can observe is something that can also exist objectively. In the material world, these diverse observable things are also disparate, but in the soul, all these potentialities of cognition are not disparate. Therefore, if we understand the nature of consciousness, then we can understand how these disparate cognitions can be unified into a singular understanding of the nature of reality. Hence, if we begin with matter, we obtain many contradictions, and if one side of the contradiction is rejected, then we get incompleteness. But if we begin with consciousness, then from the start we know about the diversities and the underlying unity.

This perfect understanding of unity and diversity is called 'intelligence', and under this understanding, we can draw inferences about the nature of the external world, which is constituted of the diversities without creating a contradiction or incompleteness. Such inferences would also be perfect knowledge about the world, because they are both consistent and complete. Thus, if the knowledge of the self is perfected, then we also obtain perfect knowledge of the world. This sūtra says that if this knowledge of the self and the world has prior been obtained by hearing, and then inferences can be drawn based on it. That hearing could be through the scriptures, the spiritual master, and so on. The implication is that instead of becoming thoughtless in order to become liberated, we can also acquire the perfect thoughtfulness to be liberated. Thus, the previous states of voidism are contrasted to the state of perfect cognition.

Sūtra 1.50
तज्जःसंस्कारोऽन्यसंस्कारप्रतिबिन्धी
tajjaḥ saṁskāro'nyasaṁskārapratibandhī

tajjaḥ—born from that; saṁskārah—the habits and impressions; any-asaṁskāra—other habits and impressions; pratibandhī—by ceasing.

TRANSLATION
Born from that (perfect intelligence) are the (true) habits and impressions, by the cessation of the other (false) habits and impression.

COMMENTARY
In an earlier sūtra, the state of thoughtlessness was described to be present with a seed from which the material life springs. Similarly, in this sūtra, the state of perfect thought is described as the seed from which spiritual life springs. The previous discussion pertained to how we can void everything, and by that it was claimed that perfection would be attained. That claim was refuted previously. This sūtra, however, says that if perfect knowledge has been acquired, then it is just like a seed from which additional thoughts spring, which then become the habits and impressions, which then lead to other thoughts and impressions, and a full-blown tree develops from the mere seed of the knowledge of the self. This knowledge, as noted above, has been acquired by perfect hearing from the spiritual master and the scriptures. When that knowledge becomes the very nature of the intellect—i.e., accepted as the perfect truth on the basis of which all other ideas are judged to be true or false—then gradually all other false ideas are destroyed by the planting of the new seed.

Sūtra 1.51
तस्यापि निरोधे सर्वनिरोधान्निर्वीजःसमाधिः
tasyāpi nirodhe sarvanirodhānnirvījaḥ samādhiḥ

tasyāpi—even those; nirodhe—in cessation; sarvanirodhān—everything else is stopped; nirvījaḥ—without a seed; samādhiḥ—similar to the origin.

TRANSLATION

Upon the cessation of even those (the false ideas), everything else is stopped, and one obtains a state without a (material) seed, similar to the origin.

COMMENTARY

Two kinds of seeds have been discussed in the previous sūtras. First, there is a material seed called the chitta, from which the rest of the material tree springs. Second, there is a seed of spiritual knowledge, or the knowledge of the self, from which the rest of knowledge springs. The additional claim is that if we plant the seed of spiritual knowledge, then it destroys the tree of material knowledge all the way to the root or the seed, and hence that state is called the (materially) seedless state. The voidism philosophy tries to enter the state of thoughtlessness which is just like the deep sleep state, while the yoga philosophy tries to enter the state of perfect thought, which is like the waking state with perfect cognition. In the deep sleep state, the root of material entanglement is not destroyed, although it becomes unmanifest. But in the perfect cognition state, the root of material entanglement is destroyed via perfect knowledge, which includes the perfect understanding of the self and of the world. However, this perfect understanding begins from the understanding of the self, rather than of the world. So, the purpose of yoga is to obtain the perfect knowledge of the self, which has been previously described to be the enlightened, energized, joyful state in which the soul calls out the Lord's name in a devoted mood.

From these sūtras we can understand that there are two kinds of yoga philosophies—one that is prevalent in the Vedic system, and the other that is found in systems pursuant to the Buddhist philosophies. These two kinds of systems are prevalent even today; even the Buddhist schools talk about meditation, mind control, thoughtlessness, and attainment of perfection through that. For the newcomer, the distinction between these two systems can be very difficult. And from the description of these sūtras, we can conclude that this difference between these two schools of meditation has existed for a very long time indeed. Therefore, after describing the perfected nature of the soul, an elaborate discussion about the differences between these two schools is undertaken.

Chapter 2

Sūtra 2.1

तपस्स्वाध्यायेश्वरप्रणिधानानि क्रियायोगः

tapaḥsvādhyāyeśvarapraṇidhānāni kriyāyogaḥ

tapah—austerity; svādhyāya—regular self-practice (which can include the chanting of the Lord's names, the studying of scriptures, etc.); īśvara—the Lord; praṇidhānāni—in complete devotion; kriyāyogaḥ—is called kriya-yoga.

TRANSLATION

Austerity, regular self-practice (which includes the chanting of the Lord's names, the studying of scriptures, etc.), in complete devotion to the Lord, is called kriya-yoga.

COMMENTARY

The previous chapter noted that devotion to the Lord is the symptom of the perfected yogi. This chapter begins by noting that the chanting of the Lord's names, the regular study of scriptures, in devotion to the Lord are also the methods for practicing yoga. Again, thus far, there is no mention of exercises as the primary practice of yoga. The lowest-level understanding described thus far has been cessations of the materialistic tendencies of the chitta. The realization of the perfect truth within a pure intellect is an even higher-level description. And the nature of the soul, and its devotion to the Lord, are the next level descriptions. Finally, devotion to the Lord by the chanting of names is the process by which the chitta is silenced, the true nature of the soul is realized, and the knowledge of the Absolute Truth is represented in a person's awareness.

Sūtra 2.2

समाधभिावनार्थःक्लेशतनूकरणार्थश्च

samādhibhāvanārthaḥ kleśatanūkaraṇārthaśca

samādhī—similarity to the origin; bhāvanārthaḥ—the purpose of remembrance (of the Lord); kleśa—the miseries; tanūkaraṇārtha—cessation; ca—also.

TRANSLATION

The purpose of the remembrance of the Lord is samādhī (full absorption and similarity to the origin) as well as the cessation of miseries.

COMMENTARY

The process of reincarnation is that if we develop our mindset to be of a certain type, then we obtain a life and a body according to that type. For example, a person who develops an aggressive hunter type of mentality is likely to be born again as a tiger. Someone who develops the mentality of always hurting others—even if they are feeding and serving us—is likely to become a snake. Likewise, if we develop the mindset of becoming a devotee of the Lord, then we obtain a life and body that is just like the Lord. This is the meaning of saying that by remembering the Lord, we become just like the Lord, and the process is not different from how by developing the tendencies of a tiger and a snake, we get those types of bodies. This sūtra also notes that when we are absorbed in the remembrance of the Lord, then all the miseries of this world are immediately destroyed. Thus, the meditation on the Lord serves the immediate purpose of freeing the soul from material miseries and the long-term purpose of taking the soul to a spiritual body in which he has become just like the Lord.

Sūtra 2.3

अवदि्यास्मतिारागद्वेषाभनिविेशाःपञ्च क्लेशाः

avidyāsmitārāgadveṣābhiniveśāḥ pañca kleśāḥ

avidya—ignorance; asmitā—egotism; raga—liking; dveṣa—disliking; abhiniveśāḥ—being invested in the body; pañca—five; kleśāḥ—miseries.

TRANSLATION

Ignorance, egotism, liking, disliking, and being invested in the body are the five miseries.

COMMENTARY

The previous sūtra stated that by meditation on the Lord, we can overcome the material miseries. This sūtra describes five such types of miseries that we can overcome. The first such misery is ignorance—which is not knowing who I am. Once we are ignorant about our real identity, we are always confused about what we must do, what choices we must make, etc. This confusion about how a person must act is the first kind of misery, and it arises due to the confusion about our true identity. The second such misery is egotism. Egotism means pride, and it causes misery because our ego is always hurt at the smallest discomfort. We think we are being insulted, mistreated, and humiliated. Then we become angry, which creates stress, anxiety, and fear, and causes even more suffering. The third kind of misery is liking, and this is a misery because we cannot always fulfill what we desire. So, we keep thinking about the various ways in which we can fulfill our desires, and without that fulfillment we feel empty and incomplete. This feeling of emptiness and incompleteness until our desires are fulfilled causes suffering. The fourth kind of misery is that we are forced to encounter situations and things that we dislike. As we are forced to deal with unpleasant situations, we become miserable. The fifth kind of misery is total identification with the body, which leads to the fear of death, old age, disease, etc. When we face these situations, we fear losing what we love the most, namely our body, and the fear of death leads to many other miseries.

When the soul becomes the devotee of the Lord, all these miseries are destroyed. For example, the misery of ignorance of identity is easily solved by the simple yardstick for making decisions—whatever is pleasing to the Lord is chosen, and whatever is displeasing to the Lord is rejected. The misery of egotism is overcome because a devotee of the Lord becomes naturally happy and satisfied, and then he doesn't feel offended, hurt, or humiliated by difficulties. The misery of unfulfilled desires disappears because the desires themselves become unimportant due to inner happiness. Likewise, even if some unpleasant situations are encountered, they become easily tolerable due to the attention being diverted toward the Lord. Finally, there is no fear of death, because the devotee knows that even if he died, he is going back to the association of the Lord.

Sūtra 2.4

अविद्या क्षेत्रमुत्तरेषां प्रसुप्ततनुविच्छिन्नोदाराणाम्

avidyā kṣetramuttareṣāṁ prasuptatanuvicchinnodārāṇām

avidyā—ignorance; kṣetram—field; uttareṣāṁ—subsequent; pra-supta—dormant; tanuvicchinna—the body is torn apart; udārāṇām—rising.

TRANSLATION

Ignorance is the field in which the subsequent (four miseries arise); they lie dormant, but on their rising, the body is torn apart.

COMMENTARY

The previous sūtra described five kinds of miseries, and this sūtra states that ignorance is the root cause of all other miseries. This ignorance pertains to not knowing who I am. In this world, we carry many identities of gender, nationality, age, race, occupation, etc. Each of these identities exert different demands on us, which are not always consistent. For example, our gender may say that we must act in one way, but our race says that we must act in another way. Then, we must act according to our age, which may contradict our race expectation. Then, there are demands exerted by our occupation, etc. In this way, we are always caught in conflicting requirements, which all seem to be part of the identity, but they are not consistent. This renders decision making very difficult, and whatever choice is made, some other identity is compromised, which results in unhappiness. The confusion about our identity leads to further problems of a hurt ego, unfulfilled desires, forced suffering, and fear of death. Thus, if the root cause of suffering is fixed, then varied types of suffering are mitigated. Thus, the import is that instead of trying to fix each of these types of miseries individually, we must fix the root issue of who we truly are.

Sūtra 2.5

अनित्याशुचिदुःखानात्मसु नित्यशुचिसुखात्मख्यातिरविद्या

anityāśuciduḥkhānātmasu nityaśucisukhātmakhyātiravidyā

anitya—temporary; aśuci—impure; duḥkha—unhappiness; anātmasu

—that which is not the self; nitya—eternal; śuci—pure; sukha—happiness; ātma—that which is the self; khyātiravidyā—is well-known as ignorance.

TRANSLATION

Taking the temporary, impure, unhappiness, and non-self as eternal, pure, happiness, and self, is well-known as ignorance.

COMMENTARY

The previous two sūtras discussed the nature of ignorance, and this sūtra further elaborates on the nature of ignorance. Real knowledge is the capacity to make correct judgments. There are three such kinds of judgments—of truth, right, and good, and these three judgments are the aspects of the self. Therefore, the first step in judging is identifying what the self is. If we cannot know who I am the we cannot decide the truth, right, or good. Once this problem is fixed, then there is the judgment of truth: anything that is temporary is untrue, and that which is eternally existent is true. Likewise, all temporary happiness is not happiness and all eternal happiness (even if it seems painful in the short run) is real happiness. This constitutes the basis of determining what is good. Finally, purity is the judgment of the right action. Whatever leads to eternal happiness is right and pure, and whatever leads to alternating misery and happiness, or long-term unhappiness is wrong and impure. Thus, the simple property of the soul being eternal leads us to the notion that truth is also eternal, therefore, the happiness of the soul must be eternal, and right action is that which leads to this eternal happiness. The process of decision making is thus simplified.

Sūtra 2.6

दृग्दर्शनशक्त्योरेकात्मतेवास्मिता

dṛgdarśanaśaktyorekātmatevāsmitā

dṛgdarśana—seeing the holes; śaktyoh—in the Lord's power; ekātmata—becoming one or oneness; eva—certainly; asmitā—pride or egoism.

TRANSLATION

Seeing the holes (discrepancies) in the Lord's power, trying to attain oneness (with the Lord) are certainly indications of pride or egotism.

COMMENTARY

In one short statement the essence of Advaita philosophy is identified and rejected. What is Advaita philosophy? It is constituted of two central ideas.

First, the material nature is called an illusion. In different variations of this idea, the material world either doesn't exist, or it exists to deliberately mislead the soul. This constitutes "seeing the holes in the Lord's power". The Sāñkhya Sūtra describes how the material energy has only one goal—namely to liberate the soul from material entanglement. The material energy is not the cause of our bondage, repeated birth and death, or any type of delusion. All these are caused by our own desires to enjoy the material world, and *facilitated* by the material energy. Advaita rests the blame of our ignorance and suffering on material energy, which is like a master who orders his servant to do something and then blames the servant for doing it. The fact is that the master would blame the servant even if the servant did not fulfill the demands of the master.

Second, the Advaita system—after blaming the material energy for all the problems—states that the soul becomes the Lord by attaining oneness with Brahman. This is even more pretentious because it now requires the notion of a fallen God. The fact is that the Lord never falls into the material entanglement, is never forced to be born or to die, and never has to suffer or be illusioned. How can the soul which undergoes all these conditions be considered God? What type of God are we talking about who is sometimes illusioned? What kind of God seems helpless and must discover his nature to find his godliness?

After noting these two ridiculous ideas in Advaita, this sūtra responds to them by stating—These are merely indications of the soul's egotism or pride. He is not able to accept that the problem lies in himself, and shifts the blame to material nature—who is the mother trying to help the child become free of suffering. And then out of pride he says that by such liberation he is now God. In short, Advaita is not even considered a responsible and mature viewpoint of the soul. It is a narcissistic idea in which responsibility is shifted elsewhere, and then a grandiose vision of the self is portrayed, disregarding the true facts.

Sūtra 2.7
सुखानुशयी रागः
sukhānuśayī rāgaḥ

sukha—happiness; anuśayī—follows from; rāgaḥ—desire or attachment.

TRANSLATION
Happiness follows from the (fulfillment) of desire or attachment.

COMMENTARY
Latent within the chitta, is another subtle body of desires and attachments, which is called *guna*. These constitute our likes and dislikes. Each person has a unique set of likes and dislikes. From the subtle body of guna, desires are naturally created due to the effect of time. Then, these desires interact with the chitta, and specific instances of previously formed impressions are instantiated. For example, some people like to eat spicy food, and desires about spicy food are automatically created in them due to the guna. However, spicy food can have many flavors—Italian, Mexican, Indian, Thai, and other cuisines. When the desire for spicy food interacts with the chitta, a particular type of spicy food desire is created. Likewise, the chitta can produce the thought for one of the many kinds of cuisines, and when it interacts with the guna, the desire for spicy dishes within that cuisine is created. These desires are like sockets or holes, and they attract forms that are exactly matched to the form of the socket or hole. When the ball meets the socket, the desire is fulfilled, and some pleasure is created. Thus, what we call 'pleasure' is the result of a ball-socket interaction.

Sūtra 2.8
दुख्खानुशयी द्वेषः
duḥkhānuśayī dveṣaḥ

duḥkha—unhappiness; anuśayī—follows from; dveṣaḥ—aversions.

TRANSLATION
Unhappiness follows from the (fulfillment) of dislikes or aversions.

COMMENTARY

Just as desires are like sockets that attract forms, similarly, if the form of the desire doesn't match the forms of the objects, or is contrary to the forms of the objects, then these objects are repelled. Just as union between a desire and its object (if the object matches the desire) creates pleasure, similarly, the union between an object and a desire (if the desire is dissimilar to the object) produces unhappiness. The objects themselves are not pleasing or displeasing. The pleasure or displeasure is the result of the interaction between an object and a desire. The material desires are always dualistic. For instance, if we like something, we tend to dislike its opposite. Sometimes, we might have opposite desires, but they manifest one after another. A non-dualistic desire is one which desires the opposites at the same time, and those objects of desire are also spiritual.

Sūtra 2.9

स्वरसवाही विदुषोऽपि तथारूढोऽभिनिवेशः

svarasavāhī viduṣo'pi tathārūḍho'bhiniveśaḥ

sva—self; rasavāhī—carrying pleasure; viduṣaḥ—wise; api—even; tathā—in the same way; ārūḍhaḥ—mounted; abhiniveśaḥ—with determination.

TRANSLATION

The wise (enjoy) the pleasure carried within the self; in the same way even those that are mounted (on the spiritual path) with determination.

COMMENTARY

After stating that attraction and revulsion to material things creates happiness and distress, this sūtra says that those who are already wise and enlightened, or those who are practicing with determination to get there, enjoy the pleasure created from the self, rather than relying on external sources of pleasure. Here an uncommon understanding of the self is presented, namely, that it itself carries pleasure. It is uncommon because we normally think that to be happy, we have to obtain pleasure from the interactions with the external world. This sūtra states that the self carries its own pleasure and hence doesn't need pleasure from the outside. Yes, there may be a need for food, clothes, shelter, etc. for the maintenance of the body, and the body is important because it helps us practice the process of spiritual realization. But beyond that there is no need for excessive consumption of needless things just to keep oneself happy. By such consumption, temporary happiness is created, but a person gets addicted to such things and is unable to live without them. Then he works day and night to procure such things, which only perpetuates the addiction. In this way, needless material enjoyment makes a person a slave to the senses. The wise and those on the path to wisdom minimize their necessities—just to keep body and soul together—in order to focus on practicing yoga. The satisfaction of spiritual practice automatically generates that inner happiness by which even a sincere practitioner foregoes unnecessary consumption of material things.

Sūtra 2.10
ते प्रतिप्रसवहेयाःसूक्ष्माः
te pratiprasavaheyāḥ sūkṣmāḥ

te—they; pratiprasava—return to the original state; heyāḥ—upon the destruction; sūkṣmāḥ—of the subtle body.

TRANSLATION
They return to the original state upon the destruction of the subtle body.

COMMENTARY
Even when some spiritual happiness is being experienced, there is always a potential for fall into the material cesspool unless the subtle body is destroyed. This subtle body, as we have discussed, comprises of desires and aversions, and these have become habits of enjoyment over many lifetimes. Even as we engage in spiritual practice, there are instances in which the past habits come back and overcome a spiritual practitioner. But one who persists with determination eventually destroys all these desires and aversions, and this is called the destruction of the subtle body. Upon this destruction, the potential for fall into material life is eliminated, and the soul attains the perfect spiritual state.

Sūtra 2.11
ध्यानहेयास्तद्वृत्तयः
dhyānaheyāstadvṛttayaḥ

dhyāna—meditation; heyas—destroyed; tadvṛttayaḥ—those modifications.

TRANSLATION
By meditation those modifications are destroyed.

COMMENTARY
In the previous chapter, the modifications of the chitta were discussed. But in this chapter an even deeper kind of modification—of desire and aversion—is discussed. Sometimes ideas from the chitta can arise, and then they trigger a desire. Sometimes, desire can arise first, and it triggers a thought. Ultimately, desire is essential for the thought to progress through the various stages of manifestation from the unconscious to the mind to the body. If a thought is produced, but there is no attraction or revulsion to it, the thought will disappear automatically. Similarly, if there is no attraction or revulsion, desires will not be created automatically and they will then not cause the production of thoughts. Thus, the removal of desires and aversions nullifies the effect of the thought modifications, and is hence considered a deeper form of purification. Even if the thoughts are purified, but the desires are not, there is always a potential for fall, because based on the desire, new ideas can always be acquired. However, if there is no desire, then even thoughts arising in the chitta are like fried seeds—i.e., they cannot fructify. With this background understanding of the role of desires, this sūtra states that meditation is the process by which the modifications of the desires are destroyed. This is different from the cessation of the thoughts in the chitta, and the key difference is as follows. By the cessation of thoughts, we can see that there is a transcendental self, different from the mind and the body. This realization propels a person on the spiritual path. But it doesn't ensure that the practitioner would not fall from the path due to past desires in the future. Hence, the reduction in the unnecessary enjoyment and keeping determination were noted in the previous sūtra. This sūtra says that if one practices meditation under such determination, even the modifications of the desires are destroyed, and the potential for a fall is totally eliminated.

Sūtra 2.12
क्लेशमूलःकर्माशयो दृष्टादृष्टजन्मवेदनीयः
kleśamūlaḥ karmāśayo dṛṣṭādṛṣṭajanmavedanīyaḥ

kleśamūlaḥ—the root of miseries; karmāśayo—the body of karma; dṛṣṭādṛṣṭa—the seer and the seen; janma—the birth; vedanīyaḥ—experience.

TRANSLATION

The body of karma is the root of miseries, of the (interaction) between the seer and the seen, the birth, and all other experiences.

COMMENTARY

As we discussed at the beginning, the soul enters the world with niyati, which comprises the past and the consequences of that past, which determine the future. The soul identifies with a past, but it doesn't understand the destiny. This destiny or niyati then creates thoughts in us and that thought is called chitta. These thoughts are then liked or disliked, which is called guna. Thus, as we have discussed, there are three aspects of the subtle body, called karma, chitta, and guna. In the last chapter, chitta was discussed, and in the previous sūtra, guna were discussed. Now, the karma is being discussed, and this sūtra states that the karma or niyati is the root of all the problems because in Sāṅkhya, chitta arises from the niyati, and prakṛti arises from the chitta. In simple terms, a destiny automatically creates thoughts in us, and those thoughts becomes desires. Now, one might ask: If the destiny is fixed, then how can the soul get liberated? And the answer is that the destiny means enjoyment or suffering, but the purpose for that enjoyment or suffering is not fixed. Therefore, we can suffer the same destiny in the path to spiritual upliftment, or in the path to material degradation. Similarly, even though destiny gives rise to some thoughts, the soul has the power of rejection—by withdrawing from those thoughts. Even when these thoughts become desires, the soul has the capacity to reject these desires—again, by withdrawing the consciousness away from them. By exercising the free won't—i.e., the power of rejection—the soul can change the *interpretation* of the destiny, even though it is unable to change the destiny.

Thus, we can think of the destiny or karma as wealth and debt, which can be spent in various ways. The wealth can be enjoyed, and the debts have to be repaid. However, the enjoyment of wealth can be adapted to acquiring the circumstances of spiritual upliftment, and the suffering of debts can be adapted to the process by which one becomes detached from the material world. Thus, by changing the use of wealth and debt, a different result is produced. There is hence a sense in which our lives are predetermined—when good karma arises, then we will automatically get thoughts and desires for enjoyment, and when bad karma arises, then we will get those thoughts which will lead to suffering. It is hence said that our suffering is a byproduct of our own choices, because a destiny creates thoughts and desires. But this predetermination in life can be changed by the soul because it has the power of rejection. Therefore, when the thoughts and desires of material enjoyment arise, then the soul can reject them. After a while, another thought and desire for spiritual upliftment will arise, and the soul can accept them. Thus, by the power of rejection of the materialistic ideas and desires, and the acceptance of the spiritual ideas and desires, our life is transformed—within the ambit of the predetermined niyati and karma.

The body of karma has good or bad consequences of previous actions. Due to good actions, our desires are fulfilled and due to bad actions, these desires are frustrated. When bad karma manifests, we cannot avoid its consequences; nobody wants misery in life, and yet, karma forcibly delivers the suffering based on prior sinful activities. The situation with happiness is somewhat different; even if there are opportunities of happiness, we can reject them. Thus, good karma gives us the choice about whether we want to enjoy. But bad karma doesn't give us this freedom—i.e., suffering must be endured. However, the interpretation of this suffering is still in the soul's control. For instance, the difficulties in yoga practice are also suffering, but we can accept them happily because we understand that this suffering leads to a fruitful outcome. On the other hand, the difficulties in material life simply deprive us of happiness. In that sense, suffering can be useful or useless. There is some useful pain and there is some useless pain. The pain endured in the pursuit of material happiness is useless pain, because it doesn't deliver permanent happiness. But the pain endured in spiritual life is useful pain because it produces a permanent result.

Thus, this sūtra echoes the same idea as present in Sāñkhya, where the root cause of the material entanglement is niyati, which is called karma here.

There is still some role for guna in determining what constitutes misery *for us*, or what we *consider* to be misery. If we enjoy spicy food, then being forced to eat spicy would be considered good, rather than bad karma. Therefore, when karma forces a good or bad situation upon us, it prior interacts with guna to determine what is pleasure or pain. If we are spiritually inclined, and we always choose the spiritual path, then even if there is some suffering due to bad karma, that helps us achieve the goals of detachment. And if there is some happiness due to good karma, then that helps us progress by additional opportunities to progress. Attachment to the opportunities to progress and detachment from the materialistic engagements become mutually self-reinforcing outcomes.

Thus, we should understand the different roles played by karma, guna, and chitta within the subtle body. Guna is our desires, karma is the deserving, and the chitta is the potentialities which can be converted into some experiences. We can also call these potentials the 'abilities' that lie dormant and are reactivated in due course of time. We cannot fulfill our desires unless there is some ability—e.g., a deaf person cannot enjoy listening to music, even if he likes music. His pleasure (and good karma) must therefore be delivered through other senses. Likewise, karma cannot act without some notion of pleasure and pain. Hence, karma is based on the chitta and the guna, and the interaction between the chitta, guna, and karma ultimately determines the type of experience.

Sūtra 2.13
सति मूले तद्वपिाको जात्यायुर्भोगाः
sati mūle tadvipāko jātyāyurbhogāḥ

sati—due to the eternal (soul); mūle—in the root; tadvipāko—those byproducts; jātyāyur—are manifest and existing; bhogāḥ—as enjoyments.

TRANSLATION
Due to the eternal (soul), those byproducts reside in the root, they are manifest and are existing as enjoyments.

COMMENTARY
After discussing the subtle body comprising chitta, guna, and karma, this sūtra says that all these become active only due to the presence of the soul. Thus, destiny is always attached to a soul. This is a contrast to Buddhism which also accepts the reality of karma, but doesn't accept the reality

of the soul. Buddhism says that destiny or karma creates an individual person, and that destiny is what causes the transmigration from one body to another, although there is no soul. This description of transmigration begs the question: How was the first karma created? If there is no choice to act, then how can good or bad karma be created? Buddhists say that karma is going on since time immemorial and we cannot trace the origin of karma. In short, our individual identity has no beginning but it has an end—when the karma is finished. Vedic philosophy also accepts that karma is going on since time immemorial, but it distinguishes between *history* and *time*. Karma is history in which one thing leads to another, and if we try to trace the cause from the effect, we do come to the point of the first event in the presently knowable history, but that first point in the knowable history is not the original point of existence in the material world because history is constantly created and destroyed. As we act in this world, a history is created; and as the consequence of our actions, a future is created. But as the karma is reaped, that history is destroyed. Thus, the Buddhist and Vedic philosophies have a similarity in the sense that both accept that we cannot trace the origin of the soul's fall because the earliest records of karma have been destroyed. The issue therefore reduces to the question of what suffering is. Can we say that some material entity is suffering? Or does that need a soul?

The Buddhists recognize that there is suffering (it is indeed the beginning of Buddhist philosophy) but they cannot explain what happiness and suffering is, or how it arises. Their claim that happiness and suffering are merely mental states is not true; there is factually a spiritual suffering which arises because we don't know who we are. When we know who we are, then suffering from the body and the mind continue, but the spiritual suffering is mitigated. In fact, a spiritually realized person can bear all the material suffering easily and is not disturbed by it. The claims of Buddhism amount to saying that there is no such spiritually realized person, which is rejected in Vedic philosophy. This *sūtra* specifically says that the karma is acting only because there is a soul. Someone is responsible for a choice, and that person who made the choice is suffering or enjoying. If that soul were absent, then there would be no pleasure or pain.

Sūtra 2.14

ते हलादपरितापफलाःपुण्यापुण्यहेतुत्वात्

te hlādaparitāpaphalāḥ puṇyāpuṇyahetutvāt

te—these; hlāda—pleasure; paritāpa—pain; phalāḥ—the results; puṇyāpuṇya—good and bad; hetutvāt—just as the causes of.

TRANSLATION

These pleasures and pains, are the results of good and bad actions, and are just like the causes of (these pleasures and pains).

COMMENTARY

This pleasure and pain are due to guna and the good and bad results are due to karma. A bad result doesn't have to cause pain; sometimes, if we see the folly in something, getting a bad result can also set us on the correct path. Likewise, a good result doesn't necessarily create happiness; sometimes, if we see the folly in the good result, then it ceases to be a source of happiness. Therefore, the good and bad results are always relative to our desires. If we change our desires, then good and bad results are both sources of spiritual perfection.

Sūtra 2.15

परिणामतापसंस्कारदुःखैर्गुणवृत्तविरोधाच्च दुःखमेव सर्वं विवेकिनः
pariṇāmatāpasaṁskāraduḥkhairguṇavṛttivirodhācca
duḥkhameva sarvaṁ vivekinaḥ

pariṇāma—results; tāpa—austerity; saṁskāra—the performance of purificatory rituals; duḥkhair—suffering; guṇa—the modes of nature; vṛtti—modifications; virodha—cessation; ca—also; duḥkham—suffering; eva—certainly; sarvam—all; vivekinaḥ—for the intelligent or discerning people.

TRANSLATION

For the intelligent or discerning people, the results of austerity and the performance of purificatory rituals are suffering, as they are the modifications of material modes; the cessation (of modifications) is certainly also suffering.

COMMENTARY

This sūtra notes how the mundane principles of morality and religiosity, such as the performance of austerity, or the development of good moral habits, are also the products of the material modes—i.e., likes and dislikes. A good example of this fact is the Varṇāśrama system in which the different classes of society such as the Brahmana, Kshatriya, Vaisya, and Sudra are defined based on their qualities, which means that each class likes to do certain types of activities, and dislikes the other activities. While certain freedom is given to each class to engage in their chosen kinds of activities, each class is also restrained in various ways. For example, the Brahmana cannot charge money for teaching or performing priestly duties; they have to beg alms and live on the offerings made by other sections of the society. This can make the life of a Brahman difficult. Similarly, even though the Kshatriya are the rulers, they cannot make whimsical or autocratic decisions; they have to be guided by the instructions of the Brahmana; this means that the rulers have to accept the mentorship of the Brahmana, which they may not like, if they are autocratic. The Vaisyas cannot break the principles of fair pricing, and cannot take undue advantage of their wealth to subvert their competition, which is difficult for them, because it restricts the accumulation of wealth. And the Sudra cannot be independent of the other sections of the society, which is difficult for them because they are denied the freedom afforded to the other sections of society (they are like the employees of the other three employers). Thus, even as everyone is granted permission to do what they are capable of doing, they are also restrained by rules and lifestyle regulations of good moral conduct. These restrictions can seem contrary to the principles of complete freedom, but they are necessary for a good social organization. Therefore, even as there is happiness derived from engagement in one's preferred proclivities, there is also distress due to the moral restrictions.

The fact is that each material mode has some deficiencies, and these deficiencies come to light when that mode becomes exclusively dominant. For example, if everyone became gentle and humble like the Brahmana, then who is going to fight the battles needed to protect the weak? If, on the other hand, everyone was fighting, then who is going to think with a cool head and propose good solutions? Thus, each mode of material nature is balanced by the other modes, but when this balancing act is performed, there is some compromise against each mode, which makes each person's life somewhat difficult, because they are not able to give free reign to the tendencies of their modes. Therefore, whether we completely stop the modifications of guna, or we permit them with some restrictions, or we give them free reign, the outcomes are always bad. If the modes are completely subverted, then nobody can do what they like to do. If they are given free reign, then society is plunged into chaos. And even if they are restricted by rules and regulations, people are not perfectly happy.

Hence, this sūtra says that the intelligent people consider all situations as painful. No material condition is a perfectly happy state of existence. We must therefore seek a spiritual existence where there is complete freedom devoid of restrictions, and yet, because that existence is based on the love of the Lord, therefore, separate principles of morality and austerity become unnecessary.

Sūtra 2.16
हेयं दुःखमनागतम्
heyaṁ duḥkhamanāgatam

heyam—ceased; duḥkham—suffering; anāgatam—not delivered.

TRANSLATION
(Austerity and purificatory rituals) do not deliver the cessation of suffering.

COMMENTARY
The mind must be peaceful to practice spiritual processes. For that peacefulness, we must stop the grossly sinful activities that lead to bad karma and constantly agitate the mind. The Vedic texts describe the principles of morality, austerity, the various rituals, etc. to minimize the accumulation of bad karma. These practices, however, do not lead to liberation, the realization of the soul's natural state of happiness, or even the realization of God. Instead, they teach us that choice comes with responsibility. Such education is necessary in a society that aspires for unlimited freedom, because the pursuit of one's desires without responsibility leads to an immoral and irresponsible society, which then magnifies the suffering, and makes it impossible to focus on spiritual goals. Therefore, even as responsible choices are always better than irresponsible choices, we should not mistake the practice of responsible choice itself as liberation. Liberation means unlimited choice and freedom, that is unconstrained by laws and regulations. This state is attained when the soul is innately happy, and

desires to serve the Lord and His devotees, without any expectations. In that state, there is no need for rules and regulations, because everything is driven by the soul's spontaneous love. The life with regulations is hence a stepping stone to the life without regulations, but we cannot prematurely disregard these regulations. We also cannot consider a life restricted by regulations as perfection itself.

Sūtra 2.17
दरष्टृदृश्ययोःसंयोगो हेयहेतुः
draṣṭṛdṛśyayoḥ saṁyogo heyahetuḥ

draṣṭṛ—the seer; dṛśya—the seen; yah—that which; saṁyogah—the union; heyahetuḥ—upon the cessation of the purpose (of the seer-seen union).

TRANSLATION

That which causes the union of the seer and the seen is perceived upon the cessation of the purpose (i.e., the goal of material enjoyment).

COMMENTARY

In an earlier sūtra, the three kinds of proofs were discussed—scriptural evidence, rational inference, and direct observation. In the preliminary stages of spiritual pursuits, we primarily rely on rational inference and scriptural evidence. For example, we previously discussed the nature of guna, karma, chitta, soul, and time, and how their interactions produce the material experience. We can understand this description based on reason. For example, we know that morality requires that bad deeds must be punished, although we cannot directly perceive the existence of karma; we only perceive it through the effects. Likewise, we cannot perceive our unconscious desires; we just know that these desires automatically manifest, so we infer that they must have existed in some form previously. Likewise, we don't see how time is acting on these realities, but by the effects—namely, that different types of belief systems automatically appear with time—we infer that these things must be caused due to time. In this way, our knowledge in the preliminary stages is obtained due to scriptural evidence and rational inference. However, when the soul is perfectly liberated, then it can perceive all these things just like we can perceive the sensations of taste, touch, smell, sound, and sight at the present. So, these descriptions are not just potential inferences that must be permanently accepted on faith. Yes, initially faith and reason are needed to practice spiritual life. But this sūtra states that once the soul has attained perfection, it sees all these things directly.

Sūtra 2.18

पुरकाशकुरयिास्थतिशिलं भूतेन्दरयिात्मकं भोगापवर्गार्थं दृश्यम्

prakāśakriyāsthitiśīlaṁ bhūtendriyātmakaṁ bhogāpavargārthaṁ dṛśyam

prakāśa—enlightenment; kriya—activity; sthiti—fixedness; śīlaṁ—virtue; bhūta—the elements; indriya—the senses; ātmakaṁ—the self; bhoga—enjoyment; apavargārtham—the desire for transcendence; dṛśyam—are seen.

TRANSLATION

Upon enlightenment, activity, fixedness, virtue, the elements and the senses of the self, the enjoyment, the desire of transcendence, are all seen.

COMMENTARY

The previous sūtra stated that upon perfection the causes of the union of the seer and the seen are understood by direct perception. This sūtra elaborates on that vision. It identifies many things that we assume based on inferences, because we cannot perceive them directly, although we can perceive their effects. Upon enlightenment, all these things are stated to be perceived directly. For example, when we perceive sense objects by our senses, then the senses move toward the objects and interact with them due to the effect of prāṇa. This movement is called kriya or activity, and the perception produced as a result of this movement is called sensation. Likewise, if the prāṇa is controlled, then the senses become fixed, and the world is no longer perceived. The movement of the prāṇa is in turn caused by lust, and the cessation of this lust causes the senses to be withdrawn and focused on spiritual activities. Now, at present we have no practical experience of this process. We cannot see how the desires push the prāṇa, we cannot see how the prāṇa is moving, how it causes the senses to move, how the sense movement causes sensations, and how simply by the curtailment of desire, we can stop all these movements. However, we can reason about these things rationally, and we can accept them based on scriptural evidence. Upon spiritual advancement, however, the soul can see how desire arises like a wave, how this wave pushes the prāṇa, how that prāṇa causes the sense movement, how that sense movement interacts with the sense objects, and how that sense object interaction produces the pleasure. Likewise, with spiritual advancement we can see how this process comes to an end. In short, whatever is gained by scriptural evidence, and rational thinking, can also be confirmed by direct experience, provided we are spiritually advanced.

Sūtra 2.19
विशेषाविशेषलिङ्गमात्रालिङ्गानि गुणपर्वाणि
viśeṣāviśeṣaliṅgamātrāliṅgāni guṇaparvāṇi

viśeṣāviśeṣa—the detailed and the abstract; liṅgamātra—merely the symbol; aliṅgāni—of those which are not the symbols; guṇa—the modes of material nature; parvāṇi—the phases or occasions.

TRANSLATION

(We also see) how the detailed and the abstract are merely the symbols of that which is not a symbol, and the occasions of the modes of material nature.

COMMENTARY

The variety of the material world comprises many kinds of details, such as the five material elements, and the abstract entities such as the senses, the mind, intellect, ego, the moral sense, and the unconscious. All this variety can be organized into an inverted-tree like conceptual hierarchy. The root of this tree is called the pradhāna, which as we have discussed, is the idea of being the boss, master, lord, or enjoyer. Everything else that follows—e.g., the moral ideals, ego, intellect, mind, senses, and the sense objects—are simply the symbolic representations of the soul trying to be the boss, lord, master, and enjoyer.

Each person tries to be the lord and master in different ways. Someone tries to prove their intellect by propounding unique philosophies; someone tries to show their wealth by building businesses; someone tries to prove their power by waging a war on others; and someone tries to show their beauty by posting their photographs on social media. All these varieties are created due to the combination of the three modes of nature. The basic bossy, dominating, and controlling mentality is divided by the three modes of nature to produce infinite varieties of greatness, and we marvel at this diversity. But a self-realized person has no such wonderment. He sees that underlying big skyscrapers, muscled bodies, weapons of warfare, or displays of wealth, there is a root problem—the insecurity that I'm not great and worthy, followed by its coverup through various kinds of dazzling displays that appear to overcome this inferiority.

This inferiority is real, and not a symbol of anything. However, the variety that follows from the attempts to coverup this inferiority are symbols of that inferiority. As a result, if the symbol is destroyed, then the inferiority returns. Thus, this sūtra says that all the symbols are created from the non-symbolic.

Sūtra 2.20
दरष्टा दृशिमात्रःशुद्धोऽपि परत्ययानुपश्यः
draṣṭā dṛśimātraḥ śuddho'pi pratyayānupaśyaḥ

draṣṭā—the seer; dṛśimātraḥ—only a witness; śuddho'pi—even though pure and perfect; pratyaya—the properties; anupaśyaḥ—observes.

TRANSLATION
The liberated soul realizes that even though the soul is pure and perfect, it has been reduced to merely the witnessing of these variegated properties.

COMMENTARY
The soul is different from the material energy, but under the bossy and dominating mentality, it is allowed to pretend that it has become great. Just like a child wears the dress of Superman or Spiderman and then runs around thinking that he has become Superman or Spiderman, similarly, the soul wears a dress that appears to be great, and he thinks that he has become great. Factually, the soul has its own greatness, but that greatness is visible in relationship to the Lord. When the soul becomes devoted to the Lord, then he performs unimaginable feats in service of the Lord, and

that is the true greatness of the soul. But when the soul abandons the service of the Lord, and tries to become an imaginary lord, then he merely observes this greatness, without himself becoming great. The result of this pretentious greatness is that no extent of wealth, power, fame, etc. truly satisfy the soul. Even the richest, most powerful, and famous people are therefore suffering from inferiority and unhappiness. Nothing ever seems fulfilling because deep within we know that even while wearing the dress of Superman, we are not Supermen. Some people who have achieved material greatness acknowledge that their greatness was a result of serendipitous circumstances or mere chance. But even that realization doesn't make them devotees of the Lord. Rather, they think that if by luck they could get this greatness, then they can stretch this luck even further. They don't know that there is true greatness in the soul, which is far more satisfying than the imaginary dressed-up appearance of greatness. The liberated soul sees this possibility and urges the materially entangled people to become the devotees of the Lord, do great things for the Lord, and thereby realize the hidden potential within.

Sūtra 2.21
तदर्थ एव दृश्यस्यात्मा
tadartha eva dṛśyasyātmā

tadartha—for that purpose; eva—certainly; dṛśya—sees; asya—his; ātmā—the self.

TRANSLATION
For that purpose (of realizing the true greatness, beyond the dressed-up appearances), certainly, the (liberated soul) sees his self or the soul.

COMMENTARY
The spiritually advanced soul sees the potential in each soul and encourages them to realize this hidden potential by becoming the devotees of the Lord. He sees this potential in himself too. He realizes that he has no limit to how much he can do for the Lord, and when this infinite potential within is realized, then the soul tries to become great by glorifying the Lord's greatness. The soul's greatness lies in its ability to glorify the Lord's greatness. This greatness can be shown through the medium

of art, science, literature, poetry, singing, etc. When we create the perfect portraits of the Lord through these media then we become great as the creators of this glorious representation of the Lord's greatness.

Sūtra 2.22
कृतार्थं प्रति नष्टमप्यनष्टं तदन्यसाधारणत्वात्
kṛtārthaṁ prati naṣṭamapyanaṣṭaṁ tadanyasādhāraṇatvāt

kṛtārthaṁ—the fulfilment of the purpose; prati—toward; naṣṭam—destroyed; api—even; anaṣṭaṁ—that which was not previously destroyed; tat—those; anya—the other; sādhāraṇatvāt—from the ordinariness.

TRANSLATION
Moving toward the fulfilment of the spiritual purpose, those other forms created from ordinariness are destroyed, even if they were not previously destroyed.

COMMENTARY
All the seemingly great people in this world are only outwardly great. If we look closer, we find that philanthropists lie, cheat, and manipulate the truth, the rich remain greedy to get even more wealth, the famous are envious of other famous people, and the powerful remain afraid of other powerful people. In all these ways, the so-called great people are quite ordinary—they have the same bad qualities as those of the people who may not be quite as rich, famous, powerful, etc. This sūtra, however, states that as one becomes a perfect soul, all forms of ordinariness—i.e., the faults in ordinary people—are completely destroyed. The term 'prati' means as one moves toward this goal. And it follows that there is continuous removal of faults and ordinariness, and establishment of all the great qualities of the extraordinary personalities. A perfect devotee of the Lord is therefore devoid of all the mundane ordinariness. He is faultless as the previous faults have gradually been destroyed by spiritual perfection.

Sūtra 2.23
स्वस्वामिशक्त्योःस्वरूपोपलब्धिहेतुःसंयोगः
svasvāmiśaktyoḥ svarūpopalabdhihetuḥ saṁyogaḥ

svasvāmi—his own master; śaktyoḥ—of power; svarūpa—one's true form; upalabdhi—obtaining; hetuḥ—the purpose; saṁyogaḥ—union.

TRANSLATION

The union (with the forms of ordinariness) is for the purpose of obtaining his master's power as one's true form.

COMMENTARY

This sūtra explains that the many faults in ordinary people are due to their desire for material mastery. The primordial material energy is called pradhāna, which means the idea of bossiness. Everyone wants to lord it over the material nature because by that lordship they think that they have become as powerful as the Lord. However, the soul is not the lord of the material energy. This sūtra states that the soul also has a Lord—the Lord of the self—and the material energy also is a servant of the same Lord, not the soul's servant. Since the material energy serves the Supreme Lord, the soul trying to imitate the Lord tries to lord it over the material energy. However, this lordship doesn't actually work. Rather, it gives the soul many types of ordinariness such as selfishness, lust, greed, pride, and fear. This is because the soul trying to lord it over the material energy factually doesn't get a control over the material energy. The material energy always remains in a superior position of control over the soul. Due to this superiority, the soul sometimes is permitted to enjoy and then forced to suffer. If the soul was truly a lord of the material energy, then it would never have to suffer. So, the soul's suffering proves that it is factually not the material energy's lord because this energy doesn't always act in accordance with our wishes. When the wishes are fulfilled, the soul doesn't remain content; it becomes greedy, lusty, and proud. This is because the wish fulfilment is not a natural thing; since it comes occasionally, and most people don't have it, therefore, the soul feels that it must be special to have obtained these things. However, there is a constant fear and apprehension that these things could be lost. Therefore, even in the pride, there is an insecurity, which proves true when the happiness is lost. Thus, all these qualities of greed, pride, selfishness, and fear make the soul very ordinary, even if has temporarily attained a powerful position. And this ordinariness begins in the desire for lordship over the material energy.

Sūtra 2.24
तस्य हेतुरविद्या
tasya heturavidyā

tasya—of that (desire to obtain power); hetuh—cause; avidyā—ignorance.

TRANSLATION
The cause of that (desire to obtain power) is ignorance.

COMMENTARY
This sūtra further traces the root of the desire of lordship over the material energy to ignorance of the soul. This ignorance pertains to the self, the Lord, and the material energy. The ignorance regarding the self is that the soul is a servant of the Lord. This was stated in the last sūtra as svasvāmi or the master of the self. The ignorance regarding the material energy is that this energy's master is also the Lord. And the ignorance regarding the Lord is that the Lord is the master of everything. For example, if the owner of a house goes out for some time, then the servant in the house may sleep in the master's bed, sit in the master's chair, or eat the food meant for the master, thinking himself temporarily to be the master. Even in this delusional state, there is a deeper understanding that the temporarily pretension of being the master is false; soon the master would return and this mastery would be lost. However, the servant thinks: Let me be the master so long as I can. Indeed, he might also desire in his heart that the master may leave the house for some time so that he can pretend to be the master. The material condition of the soul is very similar to this pretentious lording over the master's house. The soul wishes the absence of God, and demands proof: I don't see any master in the house, so there must not be any master. That means I can lord it over this house; it has become my house. The denial of its own precarious condition is the ignorance of the soul. The soul thinks that it can be happy without the Lord. Then it develops the desire to enter a world where the Lord is not visible. And it thinks that the master of the house doesn't exist, which creates the freedom to do as the soul wants.

However, as noted in the previous sūtra, this plan of independent enjoyment gives the soul many types of ordinariness, contrary to the idea of lordship. The Lord is devoid of lust, greed, pride, selfishness, and fear. The evidence that this idea of lordship is ignorance is in the results obtained through that idea. The futility of trying to become the lord of the material world proves that the idea is false. Desire for something unattainable must be rejected as ignorance. This sūtra therefore states that desire for the power of the Lord is based on the ignorance of the true nature of the Lord, the soul, and the material energy.

Thereby, the purpose of knowledge is also to understand the true nature of the soul, the material energy, and the Lord. That knowledge makes the soul a devotee of the Lord, and detaches itself from the attempts to enjoy the material world. The knowledge of the Lord is preparation to enter the spiritual world. For instance, if you were traveling to a new country, you prepare by learning their language, finding out the rules of the road, the acceptable and inacceptable forms of behavior, the weather of that country, and the appropriate clothing for it. You don't go to that country and then bumble through mistakes hoping to figure out the appropriate actions eventually. In the same way, the spiritual aspirant learns about the nature of spiritual reality to acquaint himself with that world. Likewise, the spiritual aspirant learns about the material reality to become detached from it. Those who don't understand these twin functions of spiritual and material knowledge, think that all knowledge is speculative. But that is not true; the real purpose of knowledge is becoming free from the material conditions and learning about the nature of eternal spiritual existence.

Sūtra 2.25
तदभावात्संयोगाभावो हानं तद्दृशेःकैवल्यम्
tadabhāvātsaṁyogābhāvo hānaṁ taddṛśeḥ kaivalyam

tadabhāvāt—from the absence of that (ignorance); saṁyoga—union (with the qualities of ordinariness); abhāvah—absence; hānaṁ—destruction; taddṛśeḥ—the vision of that (material world); kaivalyam—emancipation.

TRANSLATION
From the absence of that (ignorance), there is absence of the union with the qualities of ordinariness, the destruction of the vision of the material world, and emancipation.

COMMENTARY

Quite often we develop attraction for a subject after hearing about it. Similarly, we develop an aversion for something by understanding its true nature. This is the real function of knowledge—to make us averse to material nature, and to make us attracted to the spiritual nature. When this aversion to matter and attraction to spirit is acquired, then one naturally feels eager to enter the spiritual world, and exit the material world. This eagerness to get out of material existence, and to go to the spiritual world, detaches us from all mundane engagements, and upon the cessation of these engagements, the soul naturally obtains liberation—i.e., gets out of the material world. Thus, this sūtra summarizes the discussion of the last three sūtras where ordinariness was discussed, followed by the desire for lordship over the material nature, followed by its cause, namely, the ignorance of the true nature of the self, the Lord, and the material nature. Having identified ignorance as the cause of subsequent desire for lordship and ordinariness, this sūtra states that when ignorance is destroyed, then the qualities of ordinariness are destroyed (even when the soul exists in the material world) following which the vision of the material reality is also destroyed, leading to emancipation. Therefore, liberation is the result of true knowledge, and bondage in the material world is the result of ignorance.

Sūtra 2.26
विविकख्यातिरिवप्लिवा हानोपायः
vivekakhyātiraviplavā hānopāyaḥ

viveka—knowledge; khyātir—reputed to be; aviplavā—devoid of confusion or disorder; hānopāyaḥ—the method of destruction.

TRANSLATION

The knowledge that is devoid of confusion or disorder is reputed to be the method of the destruction (of the material experience).

COMMENTARY

The Vedic system comprises many books, philosophies, arguments, and descriptions. Some people wonder: Why do we need so many books? Can we not get a summary of all this? And the answer is that the summary also exists, but unless we immerse ourselves in this knowledge, we do not get detached from the material world, and do not develop an attraction to the spiritual world. Rather, those who read the short summaries without immersion, tend to spend time reading news, watching television, playing sports, or discussing politics. In short, the people who wonder why we have to read so many books don't realize that these are the antidotes to the mundane engagements in which they are already occupied, and these books can help them shift their minds onto activities by which they will develop aversion to the material world and attraction for the spiritual world. Without immersion, it is not possible to develop attraction to the spiritual life and aversion to material life. Hence, those who take their life seriously, are encouraged to immerse themselves in such books.

Sūtra 2.27
तस्य सप्तधा प्रान्तभूमिःप्रज्ञा
tasya saptadhā prāntabhūmiḥ prajñā

tasya—of that; saptadhā—seven-fold; prāntabhūmiḥ—the bounded land; prajñā—knowledge.

TRANSLATION
The knowledge of that seven-fold bounded-land (leads to destruction of material experience).

COMMENTARY
The material world is described in Sāṅkhya to be organized into a hierarchy of seven divisions. These are the knowledge of the gross material elements, the tanmātra, the senses, the mind, the intellect, the ego, and the moral sense. These seven domains are organized hierarchically from the moral sense being at the top, and the gross material elements being at the bottom. Accordingly, there are seven tiers of knowing identified even for a meditator, and the consciousness of the soul is expected to progress through these levels. The true knowledge of the gross material elements, for example, is that the body is comprised of the representations of the five sense-perceivable qualities called sound, touch, sight, taste, and smell. The tanmātra, or the sense-perceivable qualities are subdivisions within the five senses. For example, the eyes see form, color, and distance; the ears

hear tone, pitch, and form; the skin perceives hardness, heat, and roughness, etc. Then the senses combine these qualities and produce a coherent sound, touch, sight, taste, and smell. The mind then combines the percepts of the senses into object concepts such as tables and chairs, and propositions such as sentences. The intellect then combines many of these propositions into a single theory based on some axioms. The ego combines all these axioms into a single goal or purpose. And the moral sense combines many such goals into moral values such as honesty, bravery, justice, etc. If we understand this hierarchy, and their respective differences, then we can see how the soul is different from each of these. All these elements are the *contents* of consciousness, and the soul is the *consciousness* of the contents. The consciousness can exist without the contents, and vice versa. Therefore, they are distinct realities. And yet, when these contents enter consciousness, the soul thinks that it is indeed all these contents. Thus, the soul identifies with the body, the senses, the mind, and so on, and by that identification it forgets that it is separate from them. The knowledge of these realities tells us that none of these are consciousness. And by that knowledge, the soul becomes detached from material experiences.

Sūtra 2.28

योगाङ्गानुष्ठानादशुद्धिक्षये ज्ञानदीप्तिराविवेकख्यातेः

yogāṅgānuṣṭhānādaśuddhikṣaye jñānadīptirāvivekakhyāteḥ

yogāṅgānusṭhānnāt—by the discipline of yoga; aśuddhi—the impurities; kṣaye—die; jñāna—knowledge; dīptir—the light; aviveka—the ignorance; khyāteḥ—well-known.

TRANSLATION

By the discipline of yoga, the impurities die; by the light of spiritual knowledge the nature of the material ignorance is also well-known.

COMMENTARY

The previous sūtra described a seven-fold knowledge, and this sūtra speaks about the realization of that same knowledge by the practice of yoga. Yoga means union with the Lord, and when are united with the Lord, we are automatically disunited with the material energy. At that point, we can clearly see the difference between the self and what is not the self. That not-self now becomes an object, and it is clearly seen, just like we might currently see tables and chairs, and know their nature, because we do not identify with those things. Objectivity is a very important criteria for knowing the material reality, and that objectivity simply means a separation from the subject or the observer. If our consciousness is mixed-up with the content, we cannot realize how we are not the sensations, thoughts, judgments, intentions, and moral values. If we get attached to the Lord, then we can see all these things clearly as objective realities. At that point, this knowledge doesn't remain a mere theoretical viewpoint. It also becomes an experientially realized observation, just like tables and chairs. Thus, we begin with theoretical knowledge, to become convinced that we must practice yoga. And then by the practice, the theoretical is perfectly realized.

Sūtra 2.29

यमनियिमासनप्राणायामप्रत्याहारधारणाध्यानसमाधयोऽष्टावङ्गानि

yamaniyamāsanaprāṇāyāmapratyāhāra
dhāraṇādhyānasamādhayo'ṣṭāvaṅgāni

yama—what we should not do; niyama—what we should regularly do; āsana—the postures; prāṇāyāma—the regulation of the prāṇa; pratyāhāra—the withdrawing of consciousness; dhāraṇā—the fixity of concentration; dhyāna—the meditation on that impression; samādhayaḥ—full absorption in that impression; aṣṭau—eight-fold; aṅgāni—limbs.

TRANSLATION

Yama (what we should not do), Niyama (what we should regularly do), Āsana (sitting in postures), Prāṇāyāma (the regulation of the prāṇa), Pratyāhāra (the withdrawing of consciousness), Dhāraṇā (the fixity of concentration), Dhyāna (the meditation on that impression), Samādhayah (full absorption in that impression), are the eight-fold limbs of yoga practice.

COMMENTARY

The previous sūtra stated that by the practice of yoga, the seven-fold knowledge is practically realized. This sūtra identifies an eight-step process for the practice of yoga. The process begins by defining what we should not do (e.g., indulge in sinful activities), and what we should regularly do (i.e., inculcate good habits). We can call these the don'ts and do's of yoga. Most people following the yoga practice in modern time almost completely forego these two steps. For example, one of the don'ts of yoga is sex. Most people practicing yoga at present, on the other hand, use this practice to have more enjoyable sex. Such practices are clearly the perversion of the yoga system, and that means that even if subsequent steps are performed, their results are never attained. Due to the stringent do's and don'ts, the practice of this system is difficult in this age.

Sūtra 2.30

अहिंसासत्यास्तेयब्रह्मचर्यापरिग्रिहा यमाः

ahiṁsāsatyāsteyabrahmacaryāparigrahā yamāḥ

ahiṁsā—non-violence; satya—truthfulness; asteya—honesty; brahmacarya—celibacy; aparigrahā—frugality; yamāḥ—are the Yama.

TRANSLATION

Non-violence, truthfulness, honesty, celibacy, and frugality are the Yama.

COMMENTARY

Spiritual pursuits require a simple and peaceful living. This sūtra prescribes the five conditions of this living, which are called Yama. Non-violence means not hurting other living entities, and this includes abstinence from meat eating, cutting trees and forests, or generally waging wars. Truthfulness means that we don't read or speak fictional stories, apart from the obvious implication of not lying. Honesty means that whatever comes to us without cheating others is accepted. Celibacy means abstinence from sex, even using sex as a method of emotional satisfaction. Frugality means that we do not accumulate unnecessary material things, which also means that we don't spend time in earning wealth that could be used for such consumption. Only whatever is necessary for keeping body and soul together is accepted—if it is earned through honest means.

Sūtra 2.31
जातिदेशकालसमयानवच्छिन्नाःसार्वभौमा महाव्रतम्
jātideśakālasamayānavacchinnāḥ sārvabhaumā mahāvratam

jāti—class; deśa—place; kāla—time; samay—custom; anavacchinnāḥ—unrestricted; sārvabhaumā—universal; mahāvratam—the great vows.

TRANSLATION
(These Yama) are universally considered and great vows if they are unrestricted by the conditions of class, place, time, or custom.

COMMENTARY
There are certain conditions in which the aforementioned restrictions could be violated in some specific conditions. For example, one may indulge in sex to procreate. One may sometimes not refuse wealth that is automatically coming to a person, even though it is more than needed to maintain life. One might sometimes indulge in violence in order to defend one's life. One might sometimes tell a small lie to protect a greater truth. Or, one might sometimes be dishonest against a person who is even more dishonest. These kinds of exceptions are generally permitted, based on class, time, place, or regulations. However, such permissiveness often opens the doors to a less strict lifestyle. Therefore, this sūtra recommends that a person must take very stringent vows that are not broken by the ordinary considerations of time, place, situation, rule, etc. This can mean a complete abstinence from sex, strictly rejecting all unnecessary things not required to keep body and soul together, not indulging in violence even if it threatens our life, never being dishonest with others even if they are dishonest toward us, and never uttering a lie even if it can harm us. When such strict vows are accepted, then they are designated "the great vows" of Yama.

Sūtra 2.32
शौचसन्तोषतपःस्वाध्यायेश्वरप्रणिधानानि नियमाः
śaucasantoṣatapaḥsvādhyāyeśvarapraṇidhānāni niyamāḥ

śauca—cleanliness; santoṣa—satisfaction; tapaḥ—austerity; svādhya—study of scriptures; īśvarapraṇidhānāni—devotion to the Supreme Lord; niyamāḥ—are the Niyama.

TRANSLATION

Cleanliness, satisfaction, austerity, the study of scriptures, and devotion to the Lord, are the Niyama, or things that one must practice regularly.

COMMENTARY

Under the Yama, it was stated that one must not accumulate things more than necessary. However, a person can lead a frugal life, but still desire to live a life of opulence. This sūtra says that we must remain mentally contented. Cleanliness is not just bodily, but also mental—e.g., freedom from lust, greed, pride, jealousy, etc. Austerity is the voluntary acceptance of purificatory processes like fasting, waking up early, tolerating the extremes of weather, etc. Then, one must regularly study the scriptures to remind ourselves of the purpose of life, the nature of the material world, and the perfection of spirituality. Finally, one must practice a complete surrender and dependence on the Lord. Even if our mind is sometimes agitated, and we are unable to bear the difficulties of life, our body is sick, or we don't have enough to live easily, we must be assured that the Lord is always protecting us from dangerous conditions. Hence, there is no need to feel isolated or lonely, since the Lord is with us.

Sūtra 2.33

वतिर्कबाधने प्रतपिक्षभावनम्
vitarkabādhane pratipakṣabhāvanam

vitarka—contrary arguments; bādhane—in the restrictions; pratipa-kṣa—considering every aspect; bhāvanam—in a contemplative mood.

TRANSLATION

One must entertain (in their mind) the arguments which are contrary in the restrictions, evaluating every aspect carefully in a contemplative mood.

COMMENTARY

Even as one practices spiritual life, there are many doubts and contrary arguments that come up frequently. For example, we might have doubts about whether the soul and God even exist. We might doubt whether life should not be enjoyed more fully instead of performing sacrifices and austerities. We might have doubts about the rationale of restrictions and regulations, and the purpose that they serve. And we might encounter alternative philosophical positions that contradict the devotion to the Lord. This sūtra states that we should not fanatically reject such doubts, nor should we blindly accept every criticism. Rather, we must carefully evaluate such contrarian arguments and doubts in a contemplative mood, since by careful evaluation our conviction increases.

Sūtra 2.34

वतिर्का हसिादयःकृतकारितानुमोदिता लोभकरोधमोहपूर्वका
मृदुमध्याधमिात्रा दुखाज्आनानन्तफला इतिप्रतिपिक्षभावनम्

vitarkā himsādayaḥ kṛtakāritānumoditā lobhakrodhamohapūrvakā
mṛdumadhyādhimātrā duḥkhājñānānantaphalā iti
pratipakṣabhāvanam

vitarkā—contrarian arguments; himsādayaḥ—the harm they can produce, kṛta—the doer; kārita—getting done; anumoditā—in a pleasing mood; lobha—greed; krodha—anger; moha—confusion; pūrvakā—preceded with; mṛdu—soft; madhya—in the middle; adhimātrā—excessive; duḥkha—painful; ajñānān—of ignorance; antaphalā—the ultimate result; iti—thus; pratipakṣa—every aspect; bhāvanam—is careful consideration.

TRANSLATION

The careful consideration of every aspect means evaluating what harm the contrarian arguments can produce, whether they are created by us, or by the others, whether these arguments are preceded by a pleasing mood, or due to greed, anger, or confusion, whether they are too soft, too excessive, or in the middle, and whether they ultimately produce the results of ignorance and suffering.

COMMENTARY

A contrarian argument can be analyzed in many ways. First, we can identify the assumptions underlying the argument. Second, we can analyze the mood of the person making that argument. Third, we can analyze the results produced as a result of following the argument. The Vedic system of knowledge doesn't accept anything based on faith. Even if scriptures are considered the word of God, they must be carefully ana-lyzed from various perspectives. This is important because whatever is accepted based on faith doesn't become a conviction unless such rational analysis is performed. Without that conviction, people either don't follow the scriptures, or they are pressured into following the scriptures, thereby creating ignorant, blind, or fanatic followers. Either way, spiritual perfec-tion is not attained, and hence the purpose of scripture is lost.

Sūtra 2.35
अहिंसाप्रतिष्ठायां तत्सन्निधौ वैरत्यागः
ahiṁsāpratiṣṭhāyāṁ tatsannidhau vairatyāgaḥ

ahiṁsā—non-violence; pratiṣṭhāyāṁ—the establishment of; tatsan-nidhau—by the proximity to; vaira—enmity; tyāgaḥ—the renunciation of.

TRANSLATION
By the establishment of non-violence, or the proximity to (non-vio-lence), there is renunciation of enmity.

COMMENTARY
A spiritual aspirant is encouraged to indulge in contrarian thought processes, the analysis of counterarguments, etc. but discouraged from treating the person who makes such counterarguments or has contrarian viewpoints as an enemy. When faced with contrarian challenges, most people tend to become angry, as they perceive that the person arguing against them is mocking their views, etc. Thus, entertaining such contrar-ian views can lead to conflicts. Many proponents of religion get angry and violent if their religious beliefs are questioned, or subjected to rational scrutiny. As a result, they are unable to discuss their beliefs rationally, and without such questioning there is no conviction to renounce the material world, or develop an attraction to the spiritual world. Therefore, contrar-ian thinking cannot be abandoned; however, along with such contrarian thinking we must abandon the mindset of friends and enemies.

Sūtra 2.36
सत्यप्रतिष्ठायां क्रियाफलाश्रयत्वम्
satyapratiṣṭhāyāṁ kriyāphalāśrayatvam

satyapratiṣṭhāyāṁ—on the establishment of truth; kriyāphalāśrayat-vam—there is faith in the results of the actions.

TRANSLATION
Upon the establishment of truth (by contrarian arguments and renunciation of enmity), there is natural faith in the results of the actions.

COMMENTARY
The process of yoga can be long and difficult, and it must be so because it delivers the highest perfection. The greatest benefits are obtained only if we are prepared to invest the utmost commitment into it. Since the process is long and difficult, therefore, the yogi must be fully convinced to invest continuous effort. Many spiritual aspirants who don't invest the time in convincing themselves, are afraid of the difficulties, sacrifices, and tribulations of yoga, and remain attached to an easy life, even as they appear to be on the spiritual path. A true spiritual aspirant, instead, dedicates his life to continuous spiritual pursuits, even if there are difficulties, because he has convinced himself of the philosophy through proper reasoning and contrarian arguments. The person who invests continuous focus and efforts, obtains the results quickly. But those who aren't convinced, stop and start, and undergo slow progressive development, because they do not have the commitment due to the absence of conviction.

Sūtra 2.37
अस्तेयप्रतिष्ठायां सर्वरत्नोपस्थानम्
asteyapratiṣṭhāyāṁ sarvaratnopasthānam

asteya—honesty; pratiṣṭhāyāṁ—on the establishment of; sarva—all; ratna—jewels; upasthānam—are like stool.

TRANSLATION
On the establishment of honesty, all jewels are like stool.

COMMENTARY

When the sense objects interact with the senses, they can generate a desire for the sense object in us. Thus, in one form, detachment is viewed as forced separation from the objects, so that they do not trigger material desires in us. But this is for the person who hasn't yet developed honesty, which was earlier stated to be one of the Yama. If honesty is firmly established, then the attraction to such objects is completely destroyed. This sūtra says that all these sense objects—even if they are jewels—becomes just as abominable as stools.

Sūtra 2.38

ब्रह्मचर्यप्रतिष्ठायां वीर्यलाभः
brahmacaryapratiṣṭhāyāṁ vīryalābhaḥ

brahmacarya—celibacy; pratiṣṭhāyāṁ—on the establishment of; vīrya—the virility, vitality, semen; lābhaḥ—is accumulated.

TRANSLATION

On the establishment of celibacy, the virility or vitality is accumulated.

COMMENTARY

The term 'virya' indicates vitality, virility, and semen. The Ayurveda system describes the body as seven layers, in which the 'virya' is the innermost layer, and it is covered by the layer of bones, blood, flesh, skin, etc. In Sāñkhya, these 'inner' realities are described as the causes of the outer realities, and they are depicted as concentric circles in a two-dimensional plane. Likewise, there are several tiers of these realities which are like many stacked two-dimensional planes. The gross body, as we have discussed, is the lowest-tier reality, above which are tanmātra, senses, mind, intellect, ego, and the moral sense. This lowest-level reality is further divided into semen as the innermost core of the body, and the other layers being like the multiple coverings of this innermost reality. The import is that even if the skin, flesh, and blood are absent, the body can still be alive just in the bones. In this regard, the story of Dadhichi is cited whose skin, flesh, and blood has been eaten by ants, but he was still alive within the bones. When Indra approached him for his bones, Dadhichi decided to leave the body, to help Indra create a most fearsome weapon—called Vajra—from these bones. Modern science has discovered the presence of stem cells within the core of the bones, which are capable of transforming into any other cell. Sometimes scientists extract these stem cells from the embryo—even before the bones are formed—and preserve them as cures against any later health problems. It is generally believed that stem cells are not produced after the child is born. However, this sūtra means that by the practice of celibacy, these stem cells are generated even during the course of life, and using them the body becomes extremely strong, healthy, and resilient to any sickness. Effectively, a yogi who has practiced celibacy for a long time becomes free of any health problems.

Sūtra 2.39
अपरिग्रिहस्थैर्ये जन्मकथन्तासम्बोधः
aparigrahasthairye janmakathantāsambodhah

aparigraha—frugality; sthairye—situated firmly in; janma—birth; kathantā—how? or why?; sambodhah—addressed.

TRANSLATION

When a person is firmly situated in frugality, he asks: How was I born? Why was I born?

COMMENTARY

As long as we are chasing material things, the questions of "Why am I here?" or "What is the purpose of life?" do not arise, because the mind is preoccupied with how to acquire material things. Only when material consumption is stopped, then the mind becomes peaceful, and in that peaceful mind, the questions such as "Who am I?" or "Why am I here?" arise. Thus, the symptom of frugality is that these questions become the most prominent questions in our mind, and all other questions of food, sex, survival, etc. become irrelevant.

Sūtra 2.40
शौचात्स्वाङ्गजुगुप्सा परैरसंसर्गः
śaucātsvāṅgajugupsā parairasaṁsargah

śaucāt—due to cleanliness; svāṅga—one's body parts; jugupsā—disgust; parair—other (bodies); asaṁsargaḥ—disconnection or dissociation.

TRANSLATION

Due to cleanliness, a disgust toward one's own body parts and a disconnection or dissociation from other bodies (is produced).

COMMENTARY

Our body is inherently unclean. Most of us cannot stand the sight of blood, urine, stools, vomit, flesh, etc. And yet, when these things are covered up by the skin, we find them quite attractive. So, an intelligent person asks: If I am already disgusted by the urine, blood, stools, vomit, flesh, etc. then why I am attracted to a bag containing all these disgusting things? Surely, the packaging cannot make something attractive if the contents of that packaging are inherently dislikable? The process of staying clean makes us cognizant of how unclean the body is. For example, if you try to clean your house, then you realize how there is dirt in very corner. If you leave it unclean, then you don't know how unclean the house is. In the same way, cleanliness makes us aware of the uncleanliness. And that awareness makes us realize the true nature of the body, namely, that is it not attractive. By this disgust toward uncleanliness, one becomes detached from the attraction toward one's own body, and the bodies of other persons.

Sūtra 2.41
सत्त्वशुद्धसौमनस्यैकाग्र्येन्द्रियजयात्मदर्शनयोग्यत्वानि च
**sattvaśuddhisaumanasyaikāgryendriyajayātmadarśanayogyatvāni
ca**

sattva—the mode of goodness; śuddhi—purification; saumanasya—satisfied mind; aikāgryendriya—attentive senses; jayātma—the victorious soul; darśana—the vision; yogyatvāni—these are the qualifications; ca—also.

TRANSLATION

The mode of goodness—defined by purification, satisfied mind, attentive senses—these are also the qualifications for the vision of the victorious soul.

COMMENTARY

Under the modes of rajo-guna and tamo-guna, the soul becomes a servant of the body and the mind. The body produces the demand for food, and the soul says "I am hungry". The body produces the demand for sleep, and the soul says "I am tired". The body produces the demand for sex, and the soul says "I want enjoyment". In this way, the soul nods in agreement with the needs and wants of the body, just like a slave nods in agreement with the demands of the slave owner. Such a soul is considered defeated or conquered, because it is completely under the control of its master. To get out of this defeated state, one must practice the mode of sattva-guna. Three symptoms of this mode of goodness are noted in this sutra—purification of the body, attentive senses, and a satisfied mind. When the body, senses, and the mind are controlled in this way, then the soul regains its position of the controller, master, or supervisor of the body, senses, and mind. Hence, such a soul is called jayātma or a victorious soul.

Sūtra 2.42

सन्तोषादनुत्तमसुखलाभः

santoṣādanuttamasukhalābhaḥ

santoṣāt—by satisfaction; anuttama—unsurpassed; sukhalābhaḥ—happiness is gained.

TRANSLATION

By satisfaction, unsurpassed happiness is gained.

COMMENTARY

Most people think that happiness is the satisfaction of the senses, but they don't realize that this satisfaction begins in dissatisfaction—needs and wants. The senses create the demands, and then the body goes about fulfilling the demands of the senses. Meanwhile, the soul becomes the approving bystander to this process of dissatisfaction, hard work, and fulfilment. The sense fulfilment temporarily produces a feeling of satisfaction which we consider 'happiness'. But it is not true happiness; it is merely the cessation of material desires. So, we oscillate between the state of desiring and its absence, but never real happiness. Under the duality of material modes, we believe that the absence of suffering is indeed the true happiness. But one who has controlled the senses is no longer disturbed by their incessant demands, and he remains peaceful. This state of peacefulness is infinitely better than the one in which the body feels the need, then works to fulfill the needs, and then experiences momentary cessation of the needs. Most of the time in this so-called happiness is spent in unhappiness and hard work. The person who has a satisfied mind is able to overcome the states of unhappiness and hard work, and perpetually enjoys the state devoid of unhappiness. Hence, this state is much better than the alternative.

Sūtra 2.43
कायेन्दरयिसदिधरिशुद्धकि्षयात्तपसः
kāyendriyasiddhiraśuddhikṣayāttapasaḥ

kāyendriya—the senses and the body; siddhih—the perfection; aśuddhi—impurity; kṣayāt—from the destruction; tapasaḥ—the austerity.

TRANSLATION
From the destruction of the impurity of the senses and the body, the perfection of austerity (is known). Or, the perfection of the senses and the body is the destruction of impurity due to austerity.

COMMENTARY
The senses are the instruments of perception and action at the disposal of the soul. Their job is to provide the services for knowledge and action. But instead of providing these services to the soul, the senses start demanding their own maintenance. We can imagine a machine and its owner. The machine is supposed to do some work for the owner. But if the machine is faulty, then the machine's owner spends his time trying to repair and maintain the machine. A good machine is one that rarely, if at all, requires repair and maintenance. And a bad machine is one that is always in need for repair and maintenance. So, in the materially conditioned state, our senses are just like those machines that perform a little work, and then demand a lot of maintenance and repair. Instead of getting useful work done through such a machine, the owner of the machine spends his time just repairing and maintaining the broken machine. So, how do we fix

these broken machines? This sūtra says that if we deny the senses unnecessary gratification, then they will stop demanding incessant maintenance. Why? The answer is that our senses have habits. If we develop the habit of eating often, then the tongue demands taste frequently. But if we change the habits, and eat only two or three times a day, then the tongue gets used to it, and stops demanding food frequently. This is called the purification of the sense in which it remains a servant of the soul, rather than controlling the soul.

Sūtra 2.44
स्वाध्यायादष्टिदेवतासम्प्रयोगः
svādhyāyādiṣṭadevatāsamprayogaḥ

svādhyāya—regular study of scriptures; adiṣṭadevatā—the controlling deity; samprayogaḥ—communion.

TRANSLATION
By the regular study of scriptures, communion with the controlling deity.

COMMENTARY
The scriptures carry information about the Lord, and by reading the scriptures, we can associate with the Lord. Just like if we read books by an author, then we associate with the author's ideas—which previously existed in the author's mind. Similarly, the scriptures are ideas that exist in the Lord's mind, and by reading the scriptures, we can obtain the association with the Lord.

Sūtra 2.45
समाधसिद्धिरीश्वरप्रणिधानात्
samādhisiddhirīśvarapraṇidhānāt

samādhī—similarity to the origin; siddhih—the perfection of; īśvara-praṇidhānāt—by full devotion and surrender to the Lord.

TRANSLATION

The perfection of samādhī (similarity to the origin, or absorption in the thoughts of the Lord) is obtained by full devotion and surrender to the Lord.

COMMENTARY

The term īśvarapraṇidhān or full surrender to the Lord has been used many times. It was initially used to state that the liberated soul is devoted to the Lord. It was then used to describe how by devotion to the Lord, liberation is obtained. Now, the same term is used to describe how the perfected state of yoga is attained by devotion to the Lord. In this way, devotion to the Lord is the goal, the process for reaching the goal, and the state of those who have reached the goal. If you were thinking of traveling to some destination, then you must know what the destination is, what the route to the destination is, and finally, if others in the destination have also followed the same route. Hence, īśvarapraṇidhān is used in various statements to mean that (1) it is the destination, (2) it is the route to the destination, and (3) it is the route followed by those already in the destination. The term samādhī was previously noted as the eighth and final state of the eight-fold yoga system, and the conclusion is therefore that devotion to the Lord is indeed the perfection of yoga. All the processes, paths, or means that lead to the Lord can therefore be considered yoga. The specific yoga processes discussed here prescribe austerity, cleanliness, celibacy, etc. but they are not the only yoga systems. Ultimately, all yoga systems deliver the same results.

Sūtra 2.46
स्थिरसुखमासनम्
sthirasukhamāsanam

sthira—fixed; sukham—comfortable or pleasing; āsanam—posture.

TRANSLATION

A posture is one in which one is fixed in a comfortable or pleasing position.

COMMENTARY

Many people practice a variety of difficult and uncomfortable yoga postures and this practice has come to exclusively denote 'yoga' at present. This is not the understanding of yoga in this text. By a posture is meant two things. First, we can remain fixed in the posture for long periods of time, not merely a few seconds or minutes. Second, we can remain fixed in this way only if the posture is comfortable. The purpose of this fixed posture is that we can practice the control of prāṇa, which then controls the mind, which then leads to the formation of initial impressions, upon which we must constantly meditate, and then become fully absorbed in it. Those who practice complicated postures for a few seconds or minutes are not practicing yoga. They are merely conducting bodily exercises. The most authoritative scripture on these yoga postures is Gheranda Samhita, and it notes that there are 8,400,000 yoga postures—corresponding to the 8,400,000 species of life. Each yoga posture emulates a different animal, tree, bird, or fish. Out of these, only 32 postures are recommended for humans, and among them, the Siddha Āsana, a comfortable cross-legged posture is considered preeminent for performance of the yoga practice. Thus, those who are truly interested in yoga, should defocus from the varieties of postures, and pick one posture that they are most comfortable in. The primary requirement of a posture is to be able to make the body still for long periods of time.

Sūtra 2.47

पुरयत्नशैथिल्यानन्तसमापत्तभ्यिाम्

prayatnaśaithilyānantasamāpattibhyām

prayatna—practice or effort; śaithilya—loose, soft, languid; ananta—infinite; samāpattibhyām—from the ending of.

TRANSLATION

By practice or effort, (the body) becomes loose, soft, languid; it is as if it possesses infinite boundaries (i.e., that it is stretched all the way to infinity).

COMMENTARY

What we call the feeling of the body, is basically stress and tension in the body. When people pick up weights, or perform heavy exercises, the body becomes even more tensed. And some people enjoy this feeling of pressure and tension in the body. The yoga system is opposed to anything that makes the body more stressed. The focus of the yoga system is to make the body more relaxed, because when the body is completely relaxed, then we stop feeling the existence of the body. The body feels just like the air or empty space, and sometimes people (who have experienced this state) use the term 'weightless' to describe the body. The nature of this weightless state is that you cannot tell where the body ends. Of course, the body is still finite. But it gives the feeling that it is infinite. The sense of finiteness exists only due to the presence of stress and tension in the body. If this tension disappears due to relaxation, then a person feels as if he is floating in the air, and that his body has no limitation or boundary.

Sūtra 2.48
ततो द्वन्द्वानभिघातः
tato dvandvānabhighātaḥ

tatah—thereafter; dvand—duality; vā—moving; anabhighātaḥ—no attack.

TRANSLATION
Thereafter, there is no attack from the moving dualities.

COMMENTARY
The material nature is described in Sāṅkhya to comprise of the three modes of nature, which are constantly in a struggle for domination. This struggle for domination between the modes creates a battle, in which each mode dominates occasionally, and then it is pushed into subordination by the other modes. Through occasional domination, each mode subordinates the other modes, but struggles to come into domination again, so the body is in a constant state of flux and tension. Complete relaxation of the body is achieved when the mode of sattva-guna becomes dominant, and it reconciles the opposition between rajo-guna and tamo-guna. The tamo-guna represents resistance, inertia, or laziness. And the rajo-guna is activity, force, and passion. What we consider the experience of the body is the constant struggle between these two modes. The sattva-guna represents

calmness, restfulness, and reconciliation. Under the mode of sattva-guna, the constant battle for domination between rajo-guna and tamo-guna ends, and the body feels calm, restful, and reconciled. The purpose of the yoga-āsana is to put the body in this relaxed, soft, and languid state, whereas the purpose of the heavy exercises is to make the body active by force, which fights the inertia and laziness, but ultimately leaves the body in an agitated and tensed state, as the modes of rajas and tamas battle for domination. This sūtra states that if the yoga-āsana is practiced properly, then the duality of the rajas and tamas modes disappears, the tension arising by this duality is destroyed, and then the body is put in a state of restfulness and relaxation. This is the preliminary state of bodily relaxation. After this, the mind also must be similarly relaxed by the control of breath (which will be described subsequently).

Sūtra 2.49
तस्मन्निसति श्वासपरश्वासयोर्गतविचिच्छेदःपराणायामः
tasminsati śvāsapraśvāsayorgativicchedaḥ prāṇāyāmaḥ

tasmin—after that; sati—in sattva; śvāsa—inhalation; praśvāsayoh—exhalation; gati—movement; vicchedaḥ—separation; prāṇāyāmaḥ—is prāṇāyāma.

TRANSLATION
After that (the body) is put in the mode of sattva-guna; (thereafter), the separation of inhalation and exhalation is called prāṇāyāma.

COMMENTARY
As discussed earlier, the inhalation represents prāṇa (ingestion), and the exhalation can represent apāna (excretion) or udāna (expression). In between these two is holding the breath within, which represents samāna (digestion) and vyāna (circulation). Generally, most people just breathe-in and breathe-out, without holding the breath in. As a result, there is no clear demarcation between the five forms of prāṇa. The process of prāṇāyāma is meant to separate these five pranas, and allow each one to operate individually and separately.

The simplest method of separation is holding the breath both inside and outside. For example, a person can breathe in, then hold the breath in, then breathe out, and hold the breath out. As the breath is held inward, the prāṇa and apāna are stopped, and vyāna gets prominence. Similarly, as the breath is held outward, the prāṇa and apāna are stopped, and the samāna gets prominence. If one maintains silence during this process, and breathes through the nostrils rather than the mouth, then the udāna is totally suppressed. Thus, a simple cycle of four stages—ingestion, circulation, excretion, and digestion—is created. This is the meaning of dissection or separation of the prāṇa. Each type of prāṇa is exercised one by one, and thereby our consciousness is focused on one thing. If this cycle is perfected, then the activities of the body—namely, ingestion, digestion, circulation, and excretion—are perfectly balanced. We must note that the prāṇāyāma is practiced upon the perfection of the yoga-āsana. If the body is perfectly relaxed, then if the breath is controlled in the above manner, the five prāṇa are separated. If, however, the body is not relaxed, then even if we control the breath in above way, the five prāṇa are not separated.

Sūtra 2.50

वाह्याभ्यन्तरस्तम्भवृत्तिर्देशकालसङ्ख्याभिःपरिदृष्टो दीर्घसूक्ष्मः
vāhyābhyantarastambhavṛttirdeśakālasaṅkhyābhiḥ paridṛṣṭo
dīrghasūkṣmaḥ

vāhya—external; abhyantara—internal; stambha—holding; vṛttir—the modifications; deśa—place; kāla—time; saṅkhyābhiḥ—by number; paridṛṣṭah—the observation of; dīrgha—the long; sūkṣmaḥ—and the subtle.

TRANSLATION
The modifications of the prāṇa are external, internal, and holding; by place, time, and number, one can observe the long and the subtle.

COMMENTARY
As already noted, the inhalation represents prāṇa (ingestion), and the exhalation can represent apāna (excretion) or udāna (expression). In between these two is holding the breath outward or inward, which represents samāna (digestion) and vyāna (circulation). The difference between apāna and udāna is based on the place of exhalation—namely, the nostrils and the mouth. The difference between samāna and vyāna is based on the

place of holding—namely, the stomach and the lungs. And the prāṇa can also be divided based on the place of inhalation—namely, the nostrils and the mouth. Each of these processes of inhalation, holding, and exhalation can be increased and decreased in duration. And these can be of different types—e.g., breathing in slowly vs. breathing in suddenly; or moving the stomach or the chest while the breath is inhaled or exhaled, etc. The general principle of breath control is that if these processes are elongated (i.e., slower), then we can control the more subtle processes, and if they are shortened (i.e., faster), then we can control the more gross processes. Thus, for example, the regulation of the gross body can be achieved by a faster breathing in and out, and the regulation of the mind and even more subtle instruments can be achieved by a slower breathing in and out. Thus, the yogi begins with the control of the body, and as he obtains mastery, he slows down these processes, and by that he is able to acquire control over the mind.

Sūtra 2.51

वाह्याभ्यन्तरविषियाक्षेपी चतुर्थः

vāhyābhyantaraviṣayākṣepī caturthaḥ

vāhya—the external; abhyantara—the internal; viṣaya—the subjects; ākṣepī—transcends; caturthaḥ—the fourth.

TRANSLATION

The fourth kind of prāṇāyāma transcends the subjects of the internal and the external.

COMMENTARY

Once the mastery of the above type of prāṇāyāma is obtained, the next advancement is the ability to simultaneously breathe in and out. The advanced yogi for example can breathe in through one nostril and breathe out through another nostril simultaneously. Bhagavad-Gita 4.29 states this as follows:

apane juhvati prānam

prane 'panam tathapare

The term juhva means the 'tongue' and juhvati means 'feeding'. So, the yogi is able to 'feed' the outgoing breath into the incoming breath, because he is able to breathe in simultaneously as he is breathing out. Likewise, some yogis can breathe out simultaneously as they are breathing in, without holding the breath. This breath is like a pipe of running water—it is simultaneously going out and in, and the body is like a pipe through which the air is continuously flowing. This is the only type of prāṇāyāma noted in the Bhagavad-Gita, so it is understood to be the stage after which the process of breath control is perfected. In short, breath control means that there are no longer the stages of breathing in, breathing out, and holding. Rather, the air continuously flows through the body as if the body was merely a pipe through which the air passes in and out.

Sūtra 2.52
ततःक्षीयते प्रकाशावरणम्
tataḥ kṣīyate prakāśāvaraṇam

tataḥ—thereafter; kṣīyate—is destroyed; prakāśa—the light of knowledge; āvaraṇam—the cover or veil.

TRANSLATION
Thereafter, the veil or cover of the light of knowledge is destroyed.

COMMENTARY
The movement of the prāṇa controls the movement of the other things. In Vedic philosophy, the body is not the only thing that is moving; the senses are moving, the mind is moving, the intelligence is moving, the ego is moving, and the moral sense is moving. The problem of motion, which originated modern science, is far bigger than conceived at present. The prāṇa is like a 'force', similar to the forces of modern science, but it is not just moving the body. It is also moving the senses, mind, intellect, ego, and the moral sense. The basic process of this movement is that all the states of the body, senses, mind, intellect, ego, and moral sense, exist eternally, and the collection of all these states constitutes what we mean by 'space' in Vedic philosophy. This space is static, but the soul moves in this space due to the effect of prāṇa. Therefore, when we understand the 'force' that moves all these things, then we can see how the soul moves from one body

to another. Under that condition, we can easily understand how the soul will change its body at the time of death, and thereby the fact that the soul is distinct from the body. The soul's identification with the body is the veil that covers the soul, because the soul cannot see that its experience is *about* the body, and the soul is not the body. Just like when we experience an apple, our experience is *about* the apple, but we are not the apple. In the same way, the soul's experience of the body is *about* the body, but the soul is not the body. And this clarity comes to us when we understand how the soul is changing bodies.

When we realize that the soul is moving from one body to another, then a further development occurs. We realize that even the soul is not moving. Rather the movement is the changing connection between the soul and the body. Just like if you look at an apple and then at an orange and then at a mango, what is truly moving? The mangoes, oranges, and apples are not moving. Nor is the observer moving. Rather, the consciousness of the observer—which establishes a connection between the observer and the observed—is moving. The consciousness of the soul moves due to the movement of prāṇa. This consciousness is simply the *potentiality* of relationships, and the prāṇa converts the potentiality into a reality. As different potentialities are converted into reality, different objects appear in our consciousness, and because we identify with these impressions, we think that we are changing, when only the picture that we are seeing is changing. Hence, what we call the change of body is the prāṇa establishing a succession of relations to different realities. The potentiality for relationship is eternal, and the bodily states are eternal. However, the relationship between the soul and the body is temporary, and this change in relation is caused by the prāṇa. Thus, the preliminary realization about the bodily change is that the soul is 'carried' from one body to another. But an even deeper realization about this change is that neither the body nor the soul are moving. Only the relationship between the soul and the body—i.e., the experience is changing—and this change is caused due to the prāṇa instantiating a possibility.

The perfectional state of prāṇāyāma—in which the prāṇa constantly moves in and out of the body—gives rise to the understanding that by this movement, the soul is 'floating' from one body to another. How? To understand this idea, we can think of the movement of a train. This movement gives the appearance that wind is blowing into and out of the train, but the fact is that the wind is static and the train is moving forward. Similarly, the breath that is moving in and out is just like the wind blowing into the train, and the real movement is the change of body. The movement of the breath is created by the change of the body. The real prāṇa is that which causes the soul to change the body one after another, and that change then appears as the in and out movement of air.

So, the materialistic understanding of breath is that the body is static, and the air is going in and out. But the real understanding of breath is that the soul is moving from one body to another. This obviously indicates that the soul is not the body. This stage of realization is not self-realization. But it is the realization of the nature of bodily movement that gives rise to the understanding of the soul. Thus, if we obtain the understanding of how the succession of bodies is produced, then, by that science, we know that we are not this body. The process of prāṇāyāma gives us this understanding of the science of body change, and under that experience we feel to be floating in and out of bodies.

Sūtra 2.53
धारणासु च योग्यता मनसः
dhāraṇāsu ca yogyatā manasaḥ

dhāraṇāsu—the beginning of concentration; ca—also; yogyatā—the qualification; manasaḥ—of the mind.

TRANSLATION

The qualification for the concentration of the mind also (is created).

COMMENTARY

Now when the soul realizes that it is watching a movie of bodily change, and it can move its consciousness away from the body change, then the preliminary qualification for dhāraṇā or the concentration of the consciousness on something eternal is obtained. The control of prāṇa gives us the realization that we can move our attention to whatever we want, and then we start fixing our attention on the eternal reality rather than the temporary changing pictures. Note that this sūtra says that the 'qualification' for the concentration of the mind is developed, which means that the yoga practitioner can start the meditation. Until this point, any meditation is considered to be unqualified. In short, if the body is not relaxed and if the breath is not in control, then it is not meditation. This beginning of meditation is not its perfectional stage. Dhāraṇā is the stage of the mind when the mind is completely fixed on the object of meditation, but there is still a difference between the meditator and the object of meditation. In the subsequent stage of samādhī, even that difference between two objects is not seen; rather, the meditator becomes a part of the object of meditation. Since the meditation is performed on the Lord, therefore, the soul in samādhī, considers itself a part of the Lord. In dhāraṇā, the soul meditates on the Lord, but hasn't realized that he is also part of the Lord. Thus, there is a subtle difference between meditation *on* something, and oneself being part of that. These stages will be discussed later. This sūtra only notes the beginning of meditation.

Sūtra 2.54

स्ववषियासम्परयोगे चतितस्य स्वरूपानुकार इवेन्दरियाणां परत्याहारः

svaviṣayāsamprayoge cittasya svarūpānukāra ivendriyāṇāṁ
pratyāhāraḥ

svaviṣaya—the objects of the senses; asamprayoge—not in use by contact; cittasya—from the chitta; svarūpānukāra—the material form of the self; iva—in these; indriyāṇāṁ—the senses; pratyāhāraḥ—is pratyāhara.

TRANSLATION

The objects of the senses not being in use through contact with the chitta, and the material form of the self (not) being seen in the senses is pratyāhāra.

COMMENTARY

The material elements are organized in a hierarchy, such that the nature of the higher-level element is visible in the lower-level element. For example, if we construct a tree-like structure of all the species, then we can see how the properties of a mammal are reflected in cows, horses, dogs, cats, etc. In the same way, the senses of each person are unique and they reflect their personalities. In the Ayurveda system of medicine, a physician often asks questions like: "Do you like spicy food or sweet food?" or "What is your favorite color?" etc. By understanding these favorites at the sense perception level, they can understand the nature of the chitta and guna. In the same way, when the chitta is separated from the senses, then these qualities disappear from the senses, and the personality traits of the chitta and guna are no longer reflected in the senses. A simple consequence of this fact is that the senses no longer desire to eat a specific kind of food; they can consume any taste. Likewise, the eyes do not prefer to see a specific kind of sight; they can accept whatever sight is available. By this separation, the senses of perception become 'objective' and they are able to see the world objectively, rather than filtering them through our senses.

The pratyāhāra stage of yoga comes right after the prāṇāyāma stage, and the purpose of that stage is the ability to separate the tiers in the hierarchy of experience. We have previously discussed how the soul is separated from the material experience. But this separation of the soul from the rest of experience also percolates downward and every tier of experience is separated from the predisposed natures of guna and chitta. Then, our mind is not inclined to always think in certain ways; our intellect is not predisposed toward certain kinds of beliefs; our ego is not automatically driven to some goals; and our moral sense is not susceptible to some particular moral values over others. Effectively, our body, senses, mind, intellect, ego, and moral sense become impartial, unbiased, or unprejudiced, and, in this situation, they can see the world objectively.

<h2 style="text-align:center">Sūtra 2.55</h2>

ततःपरमा वश्यतेन्द्रयिाणाम्

tataḥ paramā vaśyatendriyāṇām

tataḥ—thereafter; paramā—the supreme; vaśyata—control; indriyāṇām—of the senses.

TRANSLATION

Thereafter, the supreme control over the senses (is obtained).

COMMENTARY

In the materially conditioned state, we don't have control over our senses, mind, intellect, ego, and the moral sense. The soul is just a silent and helpless approver to whatever is happening automatically. In fact, we cannot even tell the difference between the 'normal' and 'objective' behaviors and attitudes, and those that are distorted and modified by our guna and chitta. For instance, most people born in a particular type of society consider the behaviors of that society to be perfectly normal and use them as the benchmark for measuring other societies. They think that their worldview is the most natural and should therefore be universalized. Even individuals consider their responses to situations to be very 'natural', even if they get angry, upset, frustrated, greedy, lusty, etc.

When the chitta and guna are separated from the senses, mind, intellect, ego, and the moral sense, then a person realizes how they were controlled by their material conditioning, and whatever they thought was 'natural' was not their true nature; it was rather the product of various forms of previous material conditioning. In such a state, they can perceive accurately, think correctly, judge properly, formulate goals appropriately, and understand the right and wrong fittingly. Now, the soul obtains mastery over the body and the senses because now the senses and the mind fulfill the goals of the soul, rather than controlling the soul. The soul becomes the master of the body, instead of its servant.

CHAPTER 3

Sūtra 3.1
देशबन्धश्चित्तस्य धारणा
deśabandhaścittasya dhāraṇā

deśa—place; bandhah—fixation; ca—also; cittasya—the chitta; dhāraṇā—the concentration.

TRANSLATION
The fixation of the chitta in one place is called concentration.

COMMENTARY
The chitta, as we have discussed, comprises impressions, which then lead to thoughts. Concentration of the chitta, or dhāraṇā, is the fixing of the chitta onto one thought. This fixation of the chitta on one thought is termed as 'being in one place'. This 'place' or 'space' is a domain of thoughts or ideas. So, concentration also means holding one thought, impression, picture, form, etc. The prevention of the modifications of the chitta was stated at the beginning of this text. It was also noted subsequently that the chitta cannot be empty. This means that there cannot be many thoughts, and there cannot be zero thoughts. There has to be one thought, and the fixing of the chitta onto that one thought is the meaning of concentration. Of course, this is a method of practice, so the chitta may not remain fixed, even if we try to fix it. However, if the previous steps have been performed correctly, then the fixation of the chitta becomes easy.

Many people try to convert this 'one place' concentration to the concentration on some body part—the top of the head, the middle of the eyebrows, the tip of the nose, the region of the heart, the center of the belly, etc. Effectively, they are making these parts of the body as the thoughts of the chitta. But we cannot hold these types of concentrations for a long time. The thought that we focus upon must be interesting and fascinating, otherwise, the chitta will wander again. Therefore, to perfect this concentration, the yogi should think about the Lord, meditate on His name, form, pastimes, etc. This is the only way that the soul can factually attain concentration and stop the chitta's movement.

Sūtra 3.2
तत्र प्रत्यर्यैकतानता ध्यानम्
tatra pratyayaikatānatā dhyānam

tatra—thereafter; pratyaya—the properties; ekatānatā—of that one thing; dhyānam—is dhyāna.

TRANSLATION
Thereafter, (concentration) on the properties of that one thing is dhyāna.

COMMENTARY
The term 'pratyaya' denotes parts or properties. For example, if we are observing an apple, then the taste, color, smell, shape, etc. of the apple are both properties of the apple and the parts of the apple. This part-property equivalence arises if we think in terms of concepts. If we think physically, then parts are not properties of the whole, because there is no whole. Our perception always creates the whole-part relationships in which we sometimes focus on the whole, and then on the parts, then on the relationship between the two. So, the phase of concentration is the focus on the whole, and the next phase of dhyāna is the concentration on the parts or properties of that whole. Just like we might see the outline of a picture and then determine that it has the shape of a person's face, then we look within the outline and then see individual parts like eyes, nose, ears, mouth, etc. Then we can see inside each part, and by this process we ultimately recognize a person's face. In the same way, in the preliminary stage of concentration, we meditate on an outline, and subsequently, we meditate on the details inside that outline. In practical terms, this is described as a progression from the meditation on the Lord's name, to His form, to His qualities, to His activities. The Lord's name is the summarized representation of the Lord. His form is a more detailed understanding of the Lord. Successively, the knowledge of His qualities or personality is an even more elaborate understanding. And

then finally seeing the Lord's activities is even more detailed. In this way, the mind should be concentrated upon the Lord's names, and then then as the concentration slowly develops, the consciousness is gradually absorbed into the vision of the form, the qualities, and the activities of the Lord.

Sūtra 3.3
तदेवार्थमात्रनिर्भासं स्वरूपशून्यमिव समाधिः
tadevārthamātranirbhāsaṁ svarūpaśūnyamiva samādhiḥ

tadeva—even that; arthamātra—is meaning alone; nirbhāsaṁ—the apparent; svarūpa—the forms; śūnyam—non-existent; iva—in this way; samādhiḥ—becoming the same as the origin.

TRANSLATION

Those properties are pure meaning, (because) the apparent forms are non-existent; in this way, one becomes the same as the origin.

COMMENTARY

The impersonal philosopher says that one must meditate on the formless, which is without parts and properties. This sūtra says that the parts and properties of the truth are also the truth. These pure meanings are eternal, which means that they don't appear and disappear like the meanings of this material world. That which disappears becomes non-existent, and we can no longer consider it meaningful. Therefore, we must only meditate on that eternal reality. When the soul is fully absorbed in this meditation, it is termed as 'samādhī', which means becoming the same as the origin. What is this sameness? It is not identity. Rather, just like a travelogue describes the travel, similarly, the content of the soul's experience is identical to the content of the Lord's experience. However, just like the travelogue is not the travel, similarly, the soul is not identical to the Lord. Therefore, samādhī doesn't mean merger or identity. It rather means having the cognition of the Lord, just like the Lord knows Himself.

Sūtra 3.4
त्रयमेकत्र संयमः
trayamekatra saṁyamaḥ

trayama—the triad (of Dhāraṇā, Dhyāna, and Samādhi); ekatra—collected into one thing; saṁyamaḥ—is called saṁyama or the discipline of similarity.

TRANSLATION

The triad of Dhāraṇā, Dhyāna, and Samādhī is collectively called saṁyama or the discipline of similarity.

COMMENTARY

The last three stages of Dhāraṇā, Dhyāna, and Samādhī are distinguished in this sūtra from the previous five stages of the yoga practice. While the first five stages are meant to restrain and discipline the body (Yama, Niyama, and Āsana), the prāṇa (Prāṇāyāma), and then the mind (Pratyāhāra), the last three stages are meant for the absorption of the mind into the Lord's names, forms, qualities, and activities. If the last three stages are disregarded, then the yoga system is reduced to the practice of bodily restrains and yoga loses its meaning. If instead one directly tries to practice the last three stages, the body, senses, and the mind may remain disturbed. Therefore, every yoga system is common in the prescription of the meditation on the Lord, but the different yoga systems differ in the method of how to control the body, senses, and the mind. In jñāna-yoga, this discipline is obtained by immersion into knowledge. In karma-yoga, this discipline is obtained by immersion into the performance of duties without the expectation of results. In bhakti-yoga, this discipline is obtained by practicing the Varṇāśrama system of social organization, which borrows the Yama and Niyama from the aṣṭānga-yoga practice, the selfless performance of duties from the karma-yoga system, and the immersion into knowledge from the jnana-yoga system, and complements them by the worshiping of the Lord's deity.

The fact is that all these methods of mind and body control are good, but they are meant for people with different capacities and inclinations. Therefore, based on our capacity and inclination, we should choose any, or all, or some of the practices from the various systems of mind and body control, and ultimately focus on mediating on the Lord's names, forms, qualities, and activities.

Sūtra 3.5
तज्जयात्प्रज्ञालोकः
tajjayātprajñālokaḥ

tat—that; jayāt—from the victory; prajñālokaḥ—the world of wisdom.

TRANSLATION
From the victory of that (triad called saṁyama) there is a world of wisdom.

COMMENTARY
Note how the control of the body, senses, and the mind was described to lead a person to the understanding of how the soul is different from the body. But the meditation on the Lord is stated here to open a "world of wisdom". This is the spiritual world in which everything and everyone is wise and enlightened. There is no stupidity, evil, or ignorance in this world, because this world is attained by those who have perfected the understanding of the Lord. The Lord is Himself wisdom, and those who meditate on Him also become wise.

Sūtra 3.6
तस्य भूमषु वनियियोगः
tasya bhūmiṣu viniyogaḥ

tasya—of that; bhūmiṣu—foundation; viniyogaḥ—the engagements.

TRANSLATION
The engagements (of the first five stages) are foundations of that (goal).

COMMENTARY
Spiritual life is impossible without the discipline of the body and the mind. These disciplines can take many forms, and each yoga system describes a different set of disciplines. However, the optionality of each yoga system doesn't mean that all of these disciplines are collectively optional, and one can directly meditate on the Lord—without any mind and body discipline. Those who try for such meditation find themselves struggling to meet the goal, or remaining satisfied with a watered-down or

false version of spirituality, in which the convenient aspects are accepted, and the inconvenient aspects are rejected. When such watered-down versions are popularized, people get the false impression that they are indeed the ultimate truth and the goal. The fact is that they are just the inventions of the lazy person who could not handle the inconveniences.

Sūtra 3.7
त्रयमन्तरङ्गं पूर्वेभ्यः
trayamantaraṅgaṁ pūrvebhyaḥ

trayam—the three (Dhāraṇā, Dhyāna, and Samādhī); antaraṅgaṁ—of the internal; pūrvebhyaḥ—than the before.

TRANSLATION
The three (Dhāraṇā, Dhyāna, and Samādhī) are internal than the before.

COMMENTARY
This sūtra draws another distinction between the first five practices—i.e., Yama, Niyama, Āsana, Prāṇāyāma and Pratyāhāra—and the last three stages. The previous five practices are considered 'external', while the last three are considered 'internal'. The first five prepare the body, the senses, and the mind, for meditation on the Lord. And the last three use that preparatory foundation for perfecting the meditation. Unfortunately, in the modern yoga practices, the goal of meditation on the Lord is completely forgotten, and the preparatory techniques are picked selectively based on a person's desire or convenience, and the yoga teachers do not tell the students about what was neglected. In this way, they also commission the false notions about yoga by their omissions.

Sūtra 3.8
तदपि वहिरिङ्गं नरिवीजस्य
tadapi vahiraṅgaṁ nirvījasya

tadapi—even then; vahiraṅgaṁ—the external organs; nirvījasya—without a seed.

TRANSLATION

Even then (i.e., as Dhāraṇā, Dhyāna, and Samādhī are internal and important), the external organs (control is considered meditation) without a seed.

COMMENTARY

The 'seed' of material existence is the chitta, guna, and karma, which is called the subtle body. From this seed of subtle body expands the gendered body comprising the moral sense, ego, intellect, mind, and the senses. And from the gendered body expands the gross body. Accordingly, the purification can begin from the subtle body, expand into the gendered body, and then expand into the gross body. Alternatively, the purification can begin with the gross body, expand into the gendered body, and then expand into the subtle body. Both these types of processes are prescribed in the Vedic texts. The aṣṭānga-yoga system begins from the gross body, then proceeds into the gendered body, and then finally into the subtle body. Therefore, even though the ultimate goal is the purification of the subtle body, even the purification of the gross and gendered bodies is considered progress. Accordingly, the seeds of materialism in the gross body—e.g., uncleanliness, intoxication, sexual indulgence, dishonesty, accumulating material goods, etc.—are removed first. Then the seeds of materialism in the gendered body—e.g., the false ideas about the nature of the material world, the mundane aspirations for fame and glory in this world, or even the identification with a gender—are removed next. Ultimately, the materialism in the chitta and guna—e.g., that the purpose of life is my enjoyment—is removed. Once these seeds of materialism are removed, then the new seeds of devotion to the Lord can be planted, and they too grow from a subtle state, to a gendered stage, and finally to the gross stage. Thus, for example, after we change the conception of life to be the service of the Lord, we gradually obtain knowledge about the nature of the Lord, and finally we serve the Lord through a spiritual body. Thus, if the complete picture is kept in the mind, then every step can be seen as progression on the path to perfection. However, if the full picture is neglected, then one may acquire some good habits and qualities, but they are only used for expanding the seeds of materialism. For example, one can practice religion for the purpose of prestige, power, wealth, etc., rather than for the pleasure of the Lord. Thus, the uprooting of the seeds of materialism is as important as the planting of the spiritual seeds. Just as we remove weeds around a plant, and water the plant, similarly, we must water spirituality and uproot materialism. If both are not done, then the growth of the spiritual tree is stunted by the growth of the weeds, and we are unable to distinguish between the true spirituality vs. its contamination with various kinds of materialism.

Sūtra 3.9

व्युत्थाननिरोधसंस्कारयोरभिभवप्रादुर्भावौ निरोधक्षणचित्तान्वयो निरोधपरिणामः

vyutthānanirodhasaṁskārayorabhibhavaprādurbhāvau nirodhakṣaṇacittānvayo nirodhapariṇāmaḥ

vyutthāna—the uprising; nirodha—the restraint; saṁskārayoh—the impressions; abhibhava—overpowering; prādurbhāvau—the germination; nirodha—the restraint; kṣaṇa—a moment; citta—the chitta; anvayo—the connection; nirodha—the restraint; pariṇāmaḥ—the results.

TRANSLATION

Upon the rising (of the spiritual seed), the (existing) impressions are restrained, the germination (of new impressions) is overpowered, the momentary fluctuations of the chitta end, and the connection to the results ceases.

COMMENTARY

The previous sūtra stated how the gross body is purified first, then the gendered body is purified, and finally the subtle body is purified. This sūtra inverts that process and says that the practice of spiritual life not only destroys the preexisting seeds of materialism in the chitta, but it also prevents the formation of new impressions. Over time, the modifications of the chitta end, and the effects of these modifications on the lower levels of material existence such as the moral sense, ego, intellect, mind, senses, and the body also end. In short, we may not necessarily begin by purifying the gross and gendered bodies; we can also directly purify the subtle body and then as a result of this purification, the gendered and the gross bodies will be automatically purified. Thus, we can see that the progressive path of the aṣṭānga-yoga system can be inverted, and this inversion is accepted after describing the stages of the aṣṭānga-yoga system.

Sūtra 3.10
तस्य प्रशान्तवाहिता संस्कारात्
tasya praśāntavāhitā saṁskārāt

tasya—of that; praśāntavāhitā—carried by the peacefulness; saṁskārāt—from the impressions.

TRANSLATION
(Then) from the impressions, that (Lord) is carried by the peacefulness.

COMMENTARY
The perfect yogi captures the Lord in the heart, but this capture is not like forcibly capturing a mundane idea. It is the capture in which there is perfect peacefulness. The mundane capturing requires force, because the thing always disappears and we have to grasp it again. But the spiritual capturing is such that no effort is required, as the Lord agrees to accompany the soul always.

When the seed of the spiritual knowledge begins fructifying, then it produces leaves and fruits, but those are free of the unhappiness of this material world. The impressions formed under tamo-guna are painful because tamo-guna is the mode of sadness and hopelessness. The impressions formed under rajo-guna are painful because tamo-guna is the mode of struggle and hardship, although it has hope. The impressions formed under sattva-guna are dry and intellectual. The impressions formed by spiritual experience are enlightening without the dryness, exhilarating without the struggle, and modest without the sadness. That combination cannot exist in this world, due to the inherently contradictory nature of the material modes. All that exists in this world in a dualistic state exists in the spiritual experience without the dualism. The existence of such variety of emotions is the uniqueness of the spiritual experience.

Sūtra 3.11
सर्वार्थतैकाग्रतयोःक्षयोदयौ चित्तस्य समाधिपरिणामः
sarvārthataikāgratayoḥ kṣayodayau cittasya samādhipariṇāmaḥ

sarvārthata—all meaningfulness; ekāgratayoḥ—one-pointedness; kṣayodayau—setting and rising; cittasya—of the chitta; samādhi-pariṇāmaḥ—are the results of perfect absorption (or samādhī).

TRANSLATION

All-meaningfulness and one-pointedness, setting and rising of the chitta: these are the results of perfect absorption (or samādhī).

COMMENTARY

The Supreme Lord is One, but He has infinite qualities. When we perceive these qualities associated with the Lord, then we see both unity and diversity. The unity is that they are the properties of one person, and the diversity is that there are infinite such qualities. As we know these qualities one after another, the one-pointedness remains constant—we are always conscious of the Lord. And yet these qualities rise and set—just like waves in the ocean—one after another. But this rising and setting is unlike the meaninglessness of the material world, where the presence of one quality implies the absence of the opposite qualities, and without the co-existence of opposite qualities—such as bravery and humility, seriousness and laughter—the person remains incomplete. Perfect meaningfulness requires the coexistence of things impossible in this world. When the soul is absorbed in this experience, that is considered samādhī.

Sūtra 3.12

तततःपुनःशान्तोदितौ तुल्यप्रत्ययौ चित्तस्यैकाग्रतापरिणामः

tataḥ punaḥ śāntoditau tulyapratyayau cittasyaikāgratāpariṇāmaḥ

tataḥ—then; punaḥ—again; śānta—peacefulness; uditau—rises; tulya—comparable to; pratyayau—the parts and properties; cittasya—of the chitta; ekagrata—one-pointedness; pariṇāmaḥ—as the result of.

TRANSLATION

Then again, peacefulness rises, comparable (or similar) to the parts and properties (of the present state) of the chitta, as the result of one-pointedness.

COMMENTARY

The impersonalist thinks that if there is some diversity, then there cannot be unity, and under diversity the mind must be distracted and confused. This sūtra, however, states that the diversity arises as the result of one-pointedness. This diversity is comparable to the diversity of thoughts that we can presently perceive. But in the present state, we see diversity in *different things*—e.g., some people are knowledgeable but arrogant, and those who are humble are also ignorant. The diversity of the spiritual experience is devoid of this duality; the knowledgeable person is also humble; the brave person is also kind; and the strong person is also gentle. Thus, due to the co-existence of these qualities in the same thing, there is both diversity and oneness, and the opposition between these two—which exists in the material world—disappears. Therefore, these qualities are not like the dualistic properties seen in the material world.

Sūtra 3.13

एतेन भूतेन्दरयियु धर्मलक्षणावस्थापरिणामा व्याख्याताः

etena bhūtendriyeṣu dharmalakṣaṇāvasthāpariṇāmā vyākhyātāḥ

etena—in this way; bhūtendriyeṣu—the senses and their objects; dharma—their nature; lakṣaṇa—their symptoms; avasthā—their existence; pariṇāmā—their results; vyākhyātāḥ—are described.

TRANSLATION
In this way, the senses and their objects, their natures, their symptoms, their existence, and their results, are described.

COMMENTARY
The perfected state is not devoid of the senses and the body—as the impersonalist claims. Rather, the mutual exclusivity of opposite qualities is absent. Due to the absence of dualism in the properties, the spiritual qualities are not considered material. But the rejection of these qualities doesn't mean the non-existence of all qualities. This sūtra notes a fourfold understanding of this reality— (1) the existence of something, (2) its dharma or qualities, (3) its symptoms, and (4) the effects caused by these qualities by which we infer their existence. The symptom and the effect seem to be the same, but they are distinct as knowledge and action. For example, if you eat an apple, then the symptom of the apple is that it is red, round, and sweet, and the effect of the apple is better immunity from

diseases. When the symptoms and effects are perceived, then we say that there is a thing—e.g., an apple—with its qualities, such as red, round, and sweet. Hence, a difference between our perception and a reality is drawn—there is an objective apple, and there is the experience of the apple (the reality is not simply my experience). Likewise, a distinction between the object and its qualities is described (the world is not simply the occasions of qualities; rather there are objects to which these qualities are attached). Finally, some of these qualities (e.g., the ability in the apple to give better immunity) are inferred, while the others (e.g., the red, round, and sweet nature of the apple) are directly perceived. Thus, the senses of knowledge are used to perceive the symptoms, the senses of action are employed to use the thing, the mind combines the properties of knowledge and action, and an objective reality exists independent of the perceiver's mind, their senses of knowledge and action.

Sūtra 3.14
शान्तोदिताव्यपदेश्यधर्मानुपाती धर्मी
śāntoditāvyapadeśyadharmānupātī dharmī

śānta—peacefulness; udita—the rising or ascension; avyapadeśya—the localized; dharma—the nature; anupātī—in proper measure; dharmī—the object.

TRANSLATION
The nature of the spiritual state is that the qualities of peacefulness, rising or ascension, and localization are present in each object in the proper measure.

COMMENTARY
In the material world the three qualities—sattva, rajas, and tamas—are always dominant or subordinate. This dominant-subordinate nature of qualities entails that if one quality appears, then the others disappear. Thus, the person who is peaceful is not excited, and one who is excited is not peaceful. The person who is active cannot concentrate, but the person who can concentrate is not active. If duality is removed, then each of the qualities are present, and the presence of one quality doesn't entail the absence of the other qualities. Therefore, the same three qualities are

present even in the spiritual world, but these qualities are not dualistic or mutually exclusionary. Thus, when the scriptures say that the Lord is nirguna or "devoid of qualities", the impersonalist infers that there is no variety, no part, and no property in the Lord. The real meaning, however, is that these are not material qualities—those which are dualistic.

The spiritual state is noted here to simultaneously comprise of three qualities. The quality of peacefulness is the counterpart of sattva-guna; the quality of ascension or rising is the counterpart of rajo-guna; and the property of localization is the counterpart of tamo-guna. These three qualities are mutually contradictory in this world. For instance, if something is localized, then it cannot be rising. And if something is rising then it cannot be peaceful. The spiritual world allows the simultaneous existence of localization, rising, and peacefulness.

Sūtra 3.15

क्रमान्यत्वं परिणामान्यत्वे हेतुः

kramānyatvaṁ pariṇāmānyatve hetuḥ

krama—sequence; anyatvaṁ—the differences; pariṇāma—the results; anyatve—the differences; hetuḥ—the cause.

TRANSLATION

The differences in the sequences (of qualities) are the cause of the differences in the result.

COMMENTARY

The previous sūtra noted three different qualities, and this sūtra states that all variety is produced by sequencing these qualities in different orders. The nature of these sequences is that the previous quality in a sequence is the dominant quality, and the subsequent quality in the sequence is the subordinate quality. This idea can be understood akin to a sequence of digits, which have both face value and place value. For example, in the sequence 123, the first digit represents 100, the second digit represents 10 and the third digit represents 1. Even though this sequence looks linear, it is not truly linear due to the different place values assigned to these digits. The digit with the higher place value is the dominant digit, and that with the lower place value is the subordinate digit. The same number can therefore be expressed in an inverted tree structure.

In the quantitative system of counting, however, we cannot produce the entire inverted tree structure from a singular root. As a result, the hierarchical system of representation is ignored, and the linear system is preferred. In the system of qualitative representation, the 'balanced' state of the qualities becomes akin to zero, which then divides into three qualities that can be represented as 1, 2, and 3, and as these qualities divide further, infinite sequences of digits are created. Since the first place in the sequence is the most important, therefore, we can treat it as the 'outline' of a picture, and the successive places as the 'details' of the picture. Thereby, as we elongate the sequence, we create greater complexity, but they are details of the singular root. Ultimately there are only three qualities. In this way, the understanding of nature is not difficult. But we must develop the ability to clearly perceive these qualities in things.

Sūtra 3.16

परिणामत्रयसंयमादतीतानागतज्ञानम्

pariṇāmatrayasaṁyamādatītānāgatajñānam

pariṇāma—the results; traya—three-fold; saṁyamāt—by the spiritual discipline; atīta—the past; anāgata—the future; jñānam—knowledge.

TRANSLATION

By the spiritual discipline, the knowledge of the three-fold results of the past and the future is obtained.

COMMENTARY

The previous sūtra noted that all variety is produced by sequencing the three qualities in different orders, and that sequencing referred to what exists at a given moment in time. Different effects can be created by different sequences and all these effects are eternally *possible* or *conceivable*. By the effect of time acting on the prāṇa the soul moves from one possibility to another, thereby creating an experience. This experience is caused due to the chitta, guna, and karma, which remain unconscious and invisible, but the effects on the conscious experience are visible to us. The difference is this: If we know the unconscious, then we can see the past, present, and future. However, if we don't know this unconscious, then we can only see the effects on after another.

In short, if the cause is known, then the past, present, and future can be predicted. If instead we don't know the cause, we can still perceive the effects of that cause at a given moment. When the spiritual practice is perfected, then the soul is detached from the unconscious, and then it can see the varied types of impressions, habits of enjoyment, and the karma created in the past lives. When the guna, chitta, and karma are understood, then one can fully understand the past—because these impressions, habits, and consequences of actions were created in the past. Similarly, by knowing these impressions, habits, and consequences of actions, we can also understand their future effects.

Hence, the knowledge of the past and the future exists in the present and that existence is called the subtle body. That subtle body is unconscious, but it sequentially becomes conscious. According to this sūtra, with spiritual advancement, we can perceive the subtle body, and hence the past and the future.

Sūtra 3.17

शब्दार्थप्रत्ययानामितरेतराध्यासात्सङ्करस्तत्प्रवभिागसंयमात्सर्वभू तरुतज्ञानम्

śabdārthapratyayānāmitaretarādhyāsātsaṅkarastat
pravibhāgasaṁyamātsarvabhūtarutajñānam

śabdārtha—the words and meanings; pratyayānāma—the parts and properties; itaretara—mutual; adhyāsāt—from attachment; saṅkarastat—mixture of that; pravibhāga—separation; saṁyamāt—by spiritual discipline; sarvabhūta—all the elements; ruta—the true; jñānam—knowledge.

TRANSLATION

The words and meanings are mutually attached as the parts and properties (of each other); the separation of the mixture of that (word and meaning) by spiritual discipline leads to the true knowledge of all the elements.

COMMENTARY

To grasp the purport of this sūtra, we need to understand the three kinds of relations between words and meanings. First, the meaning represents a universal, and the word is an instantiation of that meaning. For example, the word 'cow' is the instantiation of the meaning of cow; similarly, the individual cow is like a word that instantiates the concept cow. Second, the concept cow is an instantiation of the concept mammal; in one sense, we can say that cows and tigers are part of mammal; in another sense, we can say that both cows and tigers have the property of mammal in them. Thus, in the former case, the cow is a property of a mammal, and in the latter case, the mammal is a property of the cow. Third, a knife can alternately be used as a weapon or a screwdriver in different contexts and relationships. In this case, the knife is the word, and weapon and screwdriver are the meanings of that knife. But if we formed a general class of weapons, then knife would be one of these weapons; in that case, the weapon would be the meaning, and the knife would be a word that instantiates that meaning. In this way, the same thing is sometimes a word and sometimes a meaning. This constitutes the mixing of word and meaning, and it leads to the confusion about whether something is the word or the meaning.

When this confusion arises, we lack true knowledge. For example, someone can say that there is no such thing as a mammal, because we never see mammals; we only see cows and tigers. But if we don't perceive the mammal, then we cannot group cows and tigers into a similarity class, and without this similarity we cannot explain their origins. Likewise, without the word-meaning distinction we cannot separate what a thing is in itself (e.g., a block of wood) and the meanings that it acquires contextually (e.g., that it can be used as a chair). The true understanding of reality is that it is comprised of three modes—the universal, the individual, and the contextual. For instance, there is a universal concept of cow, which instantiates into individual cows. As a result, the word 'cow' can sometimes refer to the universal, and sometimes to the individual. Likewise, the term 'cow' can also be applied to many different looking species, depending on the context, which then makes them individual cows that are part of the universal concept, although that characterization can change based on the context. Thus, by the mixing of these modes, enormous variety if produced, and we remain confused about the true nature of this reality. Spiritual discipline can lead to the clarity by which we can distinguish between these three modes, and by that distinction, we can know the true nature of the mode mixture. In other words, we can know if something is truly a cow, or just called a cow based on context. Similarly, we can know if this cow is part of a general class of things, or just the name for an individual thing that doesn't apply to other things.

Sūtra 3.18
संस्कारसाक्षात्करणात्पूर्वजातिज्ञानम्
saṁskārasākṣātkaraṇātpūrvajātijñānam

saṁskāra—the impressions; sākṣāt—direct perception; karaṇāt—from the instrument; pūrva—previously existing; jāti—class; jñānam—knowledge.

TRANSLATION

The impressions (in the chitta) are from the instruments for direct perception; as the previously existing classes (or categories), they lead to knowledge.

COMMENTARY

Sense perception gives us sensations, but the mind must classify these impressions into categories such as cows, horses, tigers, etc. To perform this classification, we must possess these concepts before the sense perception. The collection of all these primordial concepts is called 'chitta', and it constitutes the goggles through which we see the world. As we have discussed earlier, the chitta is the collection of ideals; these include our personal notions of what is an ideal man, woman, employee, happiness, country, house, car, and so on. When we perceive the world, we always compare the sense perceptions to these ideals. We classify them into a category if they are similar to the ideal form.

Thus, due to the possession of these ideal forms, the chitta is an instrument that classifies the world into categories such as cows, horses, tigers. Therefore, if the chitta doesn't have the prior formed impressions, then it cannot classify the world into categories. And yet, the chitta is the not the consciousness of the soul; it is a catalogue that classifies sense impressions into categories. The chitta therefore acts as the goggles through which we see the world. We have discussed the object-concept categories above, but that is not the only sense of ideality. We also have personalized ideal notions of shades of yellow and green, the ideal type of sweetness, the ideal smell, the ideal touch, and so on. It is based on these categories that we classify even the sense perceptions. The possession of such personal ideals is both a boon and a bane. The boon is that without these goggles of perception, there can be no knowledge. The bane is that if the googles are flawed, then all knowledge produced by them is also flawed. For example, if our ideal notion of happiness is not truly ideal, then we will spend our lives seeking that happiness, and yet never be totally happy. Likewise, if the notion of ideal food is not truly ideal, then we will consume that food but it will not nourish us appropriately. As we go through these varied experiences, we gradually modify our ideals. In one form, spiritual progression is moving the non-ideal conceptions of the ideal to their truly ideal conceptions. This is called the purification of the chitta. Once a truly ideal notion of everything is obtained, every time we perceive the world, we immediately know if it is perfect or not. We naturally reject those things that are imperfect, and we are automatically attracted to those things that are perfect. In this way, our experiences—even in this material world—are purified, and moved from the non-ideal to the ideal.

Once these goggles are completely clean, then everything is seen perfectly, as it should be. This is the state in which true knowledge is also obtained.

Sūtra 3.19

पृरत्ययस्य परचत्तिज्ञानम्

pratyayasya paracittajñānam

pratyayasya—the properties or parts; paracitta—the chitta of others; jñānam—the knowledge.

TRANSLATION

The knowledge of the properties or parts of the chitta of others (is obtained by spiritual discipline).

COMMENTARY

With the correct impressions in our chitta, we get the ability to not only understand the external world, but also other persons, and how they perceive the world. One example of this perception is that a person can understand the spiritual advancement of other people, the modes of nature that they are presently conditioned by, and what they need to do to advance further. Thus, a purified soul becomes qualified to guide others in further spiritual advancement. Conversely, those who are not so purified, are unable to perceive the true level of advancement of a spiritually advanced person because they keep interpreting the spiritually advanced person according to their imperfect goggles.

Sūtra 3.20
न च तत्सालम्बनं तस्यावषियीभूतत्वात्
na ca tatsālambanaṁ tasyāviṣayībhūtatvāt

na—not; ca—also; tat—that; sālambanaṁ—based upon; tasya—their; aviṣayī—not the objects of perception; bhūtatvāt—from like the sense-objects.

TRANSLATION
That (the perception of other's chitta) is also not based upon their (body); these are not the objects of perception just like the (perceptions obtained) from the sense-objects (i.e., the body).

COMMENTARY
All of us have some capacity to read a person's mind by observing their words, behaviors, body language, etc. This is because the effects are chitta are visible in the mind, senses, and ultimately the body, and a careful understanding of a person's behaviors and speech reveal their patterns of thinking. Such expressions, however, can be modified by training and a person can hide their true thoughts from others. Thus, this sūtra states that an advanced soul can read a person's mind—not by reading their bodily expressions, behaviors, speech, etc.—but by directly reading their thoughts, feelings, and mental states.

The mind is called the 'sixth sense' in Sāṅkhya philosophy because it has the capacity to move just like the other five senses. By this movement, the senses interact with the respective objects, gather information from these objects, and they feed it to the mind for cognition. The mind similarly can move and interact with other minds, gather information from those minds, and understand what they are thinking and feeling. Hence, a person who reads a person's mind by interpreting the bodily states can sometimes go wrong—just like we can misinterpret the words in a text. But one who reads the mind directly knows the true thoughts. Hence, many people report feeling 'totally naked' in the presence of a spiritually advanced person, because their minds are able to penetrate the various coverings of the body, senses, mind, intellect, ego, and the moral sense, and go into the deepest recesses of a person's existence to know them perfectly.

Sūtra 3.21

कायरूपसंयमात्तद्ग्राह्यशक्तिस्तिम्भे चक्षुप्रकाशासम्प्रयोगेऽन्तर्धान म्

kāyarūpasaṁyamāttadgrāhyaśaktistambhe cakṣuḥprakāśāsamprayoge'ntardhānam

kaya—the body; rūpa—forms; saṁyamāt—by discipline; tat—that; grāhyaśakti—the power of obtainment; stambhe—in the suppression; cakṣuḥ—the eyes; prakāśa—the light; asamprayoge—without using; antardhānam—the invisible.

TRANSLATION

By the discipline of the bodily forms, that power of obtainment in the suppression (of the chitta is obtained); (through that power) without using the light of the eyes, the invisible (is seen).

COMMENTARY

The power in the material energy is said to comprise five capacities in Vedic texts—thinking, feeling, willing, knowing, and acting. The acting capacity leads to the effects; the knowing capacity leads to the understanding; the willing capacity represents the acceptance of another reality; the feeling capacity is the ability to desire another reality; and the thinking capacity is the power to create novelty. Except for the acting capacity, the other capacities are dulled in the materially conditioned state. Thus, we are unable to create novel thoughts—this is seen in the fact that most people are not creative; we are unable to desire an understanding of reality— this is seen in the fact that most people are not curious about the nature of the truth; even if novelty is presented to us, we are unwilling to accept it—this is seen in the fact that even if the nature of the truth is presented, most people argue and fight with it; and even if we accept it, we are unable to comprehend it—this is seen in the fact that even if are curious about the nature of the truth, and we accept some description of this truth, we don't have the capacity to understand it fully. Only the acting capacity remains prominent, which means that the previously acquired impressions, habits, and karma keep producing effects, and we remain oblivious to these actions.

This sutra states that a spiritually advanced persons realizes the full potential in the material energy. This means that he is able to create novel thoughts, he develops the curiosity to know the reality, when novelty is presented to him, he doesn't fight it, rather, he is able to fully comprehend its nature. Thus, by the full activation of the powers in the material energy, he develops the capacity to think, desire, accept, and understand what others cannot even imagine.

Sūtra 3.22

सोपक्रमं निरुपक्रमं च कर्म तत्संयमादपरान्तज्ञानमरिष्टेभ्यो वा
sopakramam nirupakramam ca karma
tatsamyamādaparāntajñānamariṣṭebhyo vā

sopakramam—immediately manifesting; nirupakramam—manifesting later; ca—and; karma—the consequences of actions; tat—these; samyama—discipline; adi—etc.; parānta—the ultimate end; jñānam—the knowledge; ariṣṭebhyo—ignorance; vā—the separation.

TRANSLATION

The immediately manifesting and the later manifesting karma reach their final end by spiritual discipline, and separation of knowledge from ignorance.

COMMENTARY

Karma is divided into three parts, which are called sañchita, prārabdha, and kriyamāna. The kriyamāna is that karma which is manifesting right now. The prārabdha is the karma that was fixed at the time of birth, and will manifest over time in this life. And sañchita is that karma which will manifest after this life. This sūtra appears to combine the kriyamāna and prārabdha into the category called sopakramam, and the sañchita is called nirupakramam. These terms basically mean "that which is already sequenced" and "that which is not yet sequenced". Then this sūtra says that both these types of karma come to their ultimate end when perfect knowledge is obtained by spiritual discipline. The perfection of knowledge means the purification of the chitta and the guna. In short, we acquire perfect ideas and desires. Then, when no more correction to our thinking and desiring is needed, the karma comes to an end.

Sūtra 3.23
मैत्र्यादिषु बलानि
maitryādiṣu balāni

maitryādiṣu—from (the restriction) on friendship; balāni—strength.

TRANSLATION
Through the restrictions on friendships, strength is acquired.

COMMENTARY
Once the karma is destroyed, the soul restricts its 'friendships', which is another way of saying the restrains his connections to this world. By such restraint, this sūtra states, immense power is acquired. We must remember that this power is not something that we exercise on others, because we have already restrained the 'friendships' It is rather that inner strength or self-confidence about one's ability to do anything. It is a fact of life that those people who maintain social relationships are internally weak. They depend on other people being there for them and they gain strength from their presence. If these relationships disappeared, then the person would also suffer from insecurity and loneliness. The person who lives alone, instead, develops the strength to just rely on themselves, and they stop needing other people. So, the indication is that the yogi also lives alone, and by that aloofness he develops internal strength.

Sūtra 3.24
बलेषु हस्तिबलादीनि
baleṣu hastibalādīni

baleṣu—by (restrictions on) strength; hastibalādīni—strength like an elephant.

TRANSLATION

Through the restrictions on strengths, elephant-like strength is acquired.

COMMENTARY

Even as one acquires immense self-confidence and ability simply by living alone, one must further restrain the use of this strength. That strength must rather be channeled into only the necessary activities. When the growing strength is further restrained in this way, this sūtra states, the strength grows further. Ultimately, the person becomes fearless, due to the confidence in his ability. Here is a clear indication that even though a person many have immense self-confidence, he must not use this confidence for overpowering other people. If this strength is used, then again, a dependence on others is created, and that dependence further weakens a person. So, one might ask: What is the use of strength if not using it on others? The answer is that this strength is required to conquer the temptations of the material energy. Even a moment of weakness, where the soul thinks that it is incomplete, can lead it to seek fulfilment in relationships to other things. When immense strength is established, then the soul feels no need for other things, because it always remains self-fulfilled. Therefore, the strength is not for controlling the others; it is only for self-control.

Sūtra 3.25

परवृत्त्यालोकन्यासात्सूक्ष्मव्यवहतिवप्रिरकृष्टज्ञानम्

pravṛttyālokanyāsātsūkṣmavyavahitaviprakṛṣṭajñānam

pravṛtti—the tendencies; āloka—the light; anyāsāt—by non-engagement; sūkṣma—subtle; vyavahita—things that are obstructed from our vision; viprakṛṣṭa—things that are distant; jñānam—are known.

TRANSLATION

The tendencies of the chitta are illuminated by non-engagement; then, the subtle, the things obstructed from vision, and things that are distant, are known.

COMMENTARY

The chitta comprises of many layers of conditioning. As these layers are removed, new layers that were previously hidden come to light. Then we begin realizing the extent of our problem. Greater purification of the chitta, therefore, often brings us face to face with problems we did not know even existed. This can discourage the spiritual aspirant, but there is no need to panic. It is a natural outcome of progress, that much of what is subtle and unconscious, things that we did not know existed within us, and the impressions that were formed in the distant past, but remain suppressed for a long time, become visible.

In the previous sūtra, elephant-like strength was described. We can now see why this type of strength is needed—the deeper impressions are also harder to remove. The desires that we have cultivated over a long period of time have become strong habits, and we cannot give up these desires easily. Likewise, the notions of ideals that we have accepted over long periods of time have become entrenched in our unconscious. We are unable to uproot these false ideals and irresistible desires unless we develop the power to conquer the material temptations. As one gets more purified, the further purification becomes harder. Therefore, the process seems rapid in the beginning, but slow over time. To accelerate the process of purification one must develop great inner strength to conquer the deepest level false ideals and temptations of material desires.

Sūtra 3.26
भुवनज्ञानं सूर्ये संयमात्
bhuvanajñānaṁ sūrye saṁyamāt

bhuvana—the planetary systems; jñānaṁ—knowledge; sūrye—of the sun; saṁyamāt—by the regulatory practices.

TRANSLATION

The knowledge of the various planetary systems is obtained by the regulatory practices related to the sun.

COMMENTARY

Earth is not the only place life is found. There are many higher and lower planetary systems where different kinds of life forms are found. These places are described in Purana, and this sūtra states that a complete understanding of these planetary systems is obtained by the regulatory practices of the sun.

This sun, however, doesn't refer to the luminous body in the sky. Beginning with this sūtra, several centers in the body are described. The regulatory practice referred to in this sūtra (and the subsequent ones) refers to the centers in the body. Since these practices are not elaborated here, we can understand these forms of meditations as methods by which many kinds of knowledge are acquired. This sūtra says that following the regulatory practice related to the sun center in the body, the knowledge of all the planetary systems is obtained.

When we view the universe semantically, then the higher-level realities are reflected inside the lower-level realities. For example, the concept mammal is immanent in the concept cow, even though the concept mammal transcends the concept cow. We can say that the concept mammal is an object, the concept cow is a mirror, and the mammal reflected in the cow is the image. Thus, by meditating on the reflected image, we get the same knowledge as if we were seeing the real object. Furthermore, each reflected reality may in turn be reflecting other realities. For example, in this sūtra, it is indicated that the knowledge of the planetary systems is present in the sun. Therefore, we are talking about a second-order reflection—the sun reflected in our bodies, and the planetary systems reflected inside that representation of the sun. These practices are clearly meant for those who are very advanced. As the previous sūtras have discussed, a progressive path leads to the cleansing of the chitta and guna, and the destruction of karma. Once this perfection is attained, then by various meditative practices, the knowledge of the entire universe can be obtained—without going to these places. A soul who is completely purified has no desire to go to any other place, but he may be curious to know about the parts of the Lord's creation. These practices can be used to satisfy the various kinds of curiosities.

Sūtra 3.27
चन्द्रे ताराव्यूहज्ञानम्
candre tārāvyūhajñānam

candre—of the moon; tārā—the stars; vyūha—constellations; jñānam—knowledge.

TRANSLATION

The knowledge of the various star constellations is obtained by the worship or the regulatory practices related to the moon (center in the body).

COMMENTARY

Yet again, there is a moon reflection in the body, and inside that reflection there are reflections of the star constellations. Thus, by concentrating on the moon reflection, one should be able to see the star constellations. We can take these practices as the symptoms to be satisfied by the perfected aśtānga-yogi. The implication is that the entire universe is like a body, and that body is reflected in a miniature form within our body. Therefore, truly understanding our body means understanding the entire universe. This type of knowledge is obtained not by going further and further outward, but more and more inward. Thus, instead of looking into the sky to understand the nature of the universe, the yogi looks into his own body, and by that, he understands the universe.

Sūtra 3.28
ध्रुवे तद्गतज्ञानम्
dhruve tadgatijñānam

dhruve—of the pole star; tadgati—the activities (of the stars); jñānam—are known.

TRANSLATION

The knowledge of the activities of the star constellations is obtained by the worship or the regulatory practices related to the pole star (in the body).

COMMENTARY

All over the world, there are three main branches of religion—of the sun, the moon, and the stars. Based on these forms of worship, there are three prominent calendars—solar, lunar, and sidereal. These three forms of worship are extensions of the worship of Lord Viṣṇu (sun), Śiva (moon), and Brahma (stars). Hence, three forms of worship are prescribed here, but all other planets such as Jupiter, Mars, Saturn, Venus, and Mercury are not mentioned. We can take this to imply that these three are considered the most important forms of religiosity. In an earlier sūtra, it was noted that the study of the sun suffices to understand all the other planets. Likewise, the study of the moon suffices to understand all the stars. The pole star is excluded from this study, which means that it has an effect on the movements of the sun and moon as well. This process is described in Vedic cosmology where the pole star causes the movement of the zodiac, the zodiac movement then causes a 'drag' on the movement of the sun, and the sun's movement then causes a 'drag' on the moon's movement. The complex relation between these movements is not discussed here; it is just noted that a yogi obtains a full understanding of these movements by his meditation.

People new to the Vedic descriptions on cosmology sometimes ask: How did people in the past know about the universe when they did not have telescopes? The answer to that question is presented in these sūtras. Their advanced knowledge of the universe is not based on external observation. It is rather based on the understanding of the reflections of these interactions in the body. Since the body reflects everything, therefore, in one sense, we can know everything from the body itself. The yogi gains perfect knowledge in this way.

Sūtra 3.29
नाभिचक्रे कायव्यूहज्ञानम्
nābhicakre kāyavyūhajñānam

nābhicakre—the chakra of the navel; kāyavyūha—the structure of the body; jñānam—knowledge.

TRANSLATION
The knowledge of the structure of the body is obtained by the regulatory practices related to the chakra of the navel.

COMMENTARY
The body has three main centers: in the head, the heart, and the navel. The center in the head is responsible for cognition; the center in the heart is responsible for emotion; and the center in the navel is responsible for relation. We can think of these three centers as the purpose, matter, and structure. To understand this idea, we can think of a team of people. The individual persons in the team are the 'matter'. Their organization into

different functional roles is the 'structure'. And the reason for which the team exists is the 'purpose'. A team originates in the purpose, following which a functional structure is created, following which the roles in the functional structure are populated. In the same way, the region in the heart constitutes the purpose for the existence of the body; the region in the navel controls the functional structure in the body; and the region in the head controls the various parts—within their defined functionality.

This sūtra states that by focusing on the region of the navel we can understand the structure of the body. This structural component of the body defines how the different parts function, and whether they are functioning correctly. In subsequent sūtras, we will see the other two components—namely, in the head (the crown) and in the heart (where the soul is present)—also being discussed.

Sūtra 3.30

कण्ठकूपे क्षुत्पिपासानिवृत्तिः

kaṇṭhakūpe kṣutpipāsānivṛttiḥ

kaṇṭhakūpe—the cavity of the throat; kṣutpipāsā—hunger and thirst; nivṛttiḥ—cessation.

TRANSLATION

By the regulatory practices related to the cavity of the throat, there is cessation of hunger and thirst.

COMMENTARY

The regulatory practice on the navel requires that the stomach be empty—i.e., without food and water. Therefore, another regulatory practice is prescribed to overcome the feelings of hunger and thirst, and put the region of the navel to rest. These regulatory practices involve producing certain specific types of sounds, which destroy the feelings of hunger and thirst. In this regard, we can note that a general principle of all yoga practice is to avoid talking unnecessarily. In fact, if the topic isn't related to spiritual activities, one should not talk. This not only conserves the bodily energy, but also controls the mind. By regulating the speech, or by producing specific kinds of sounds, the hunger and thirst are automatically destroyed. This helps in regulating the navel chakra.

Sūtra 3.31
कूर्मनाड्यां स्थैर्यम्
kūrmanāḍyāṁ sthairyam

kūrmanāḍyāṁ—the tortoise channel (the bronchial tube); sthairyam—calmness.

TRANSLATION
By the regulatory practices of the bronchial tube, calmness is attained.

COMMENTARY
In the Ayurvedic system, a broad classification of the body divides it into three parts—the head is considered sattva-guna, the region of the heart is considered rajo-guna, and the region of the stomach is considered tamo-guna. This division of the body pertains to the different categories of emotions, and how they affect different parts of the body. The region of the stomach carries the emotions of tamo-guna—fear, anxiety, hopeless-ness, weakness, etc. The region of the heart carries the emotions of rajo-guna—love, desire, compassion, empathy, etc. Finally, the region of the head carries the emotions of sattva-guna—solitude, curiosity, satisfaction, detachment, etc. To practice any kind of concentration, one has to enter the state of sattva-guna, and this is especially true of the concentration on the navel, because it is the most restless part of the body. Therefore, another regulatory practice is described to put the navel at rest. This regulation is nothing other than prāṇāyāma, and this means that one can perform the concentration on the navel after the prāṇāyāma stage is perfected.

Sūtra 3.32
मूर्धज्योतिषि सिद्धिदर्शनम्
mūrdhajyotiṣi siddhadarśanam

mūrdhajyotiṣi—the light of the crown; siddhadarśanam—those who possess mystical powers (the siddha), or the mystical powers themselves are seen.

TRANSLATION

By the regulatory practices related to the light of the crown, those possessing the mystical powers, or the mystical powers themselves, are seen.

COMMENTARY

As discussed earlier, the body has three main centers in the head, the heart, and the navel. Previously, the center in the navel was discussed. In this sūtra, the center in the head is discussed. And in the next sūtra, the center in the heart is discussed. The center in the head is responsible for the understanding of the laws of nature. Once this understanding is obtained, there are eight kinds of mystical abilities, such as the ability to become very small or very large, to become very light or very heavy, and so forth. The knowledge of matter therefore leads to extraordinary material capabilities. In the Sāñkhya Sūtra, it is stated that these capabilities do not lead to liberation. Indeed, if they are acquired before karma, guna, and chitta are purified, they can drag a person again into material entanglement. However, for a liberated person, these capabilities are obtained automatically without a separate endeavor for them. Therefore, these statements about mystical power should not be seen as encouragement for the pursuit of such powers, but as symptoms of one who has become perfect.

Sūtra 3.33

प्रातिभाद्वा सर्वम्

prātibhādvā sarvam

prātibhāt—by the talent (acquired through spiritual practice); vā—or; sarvam—everything (can be known).

TRANSLATION

Or, by the talent acquired via spiritual practice, everything can be known.

COMMENTARY

Finally, we come to the meditation in the heart (this point will be further clarified in the next sūtra, where the heart is mentioned), which is said to reveal everything. This is because we are no longer relying on our bodily abilities to know. Instead, we rely on the Paramātma in the heart to give us all knowledge. As discussed in previous sūtras, there are various practices by which one can conquer hunger and thirst, or even obtain various mystical abilities. This sūtra, however, states that one who has obtained spiritual perfection automatically obtains all the mystical powers, overcomes the anxiety and fears, and obtains control over the bodily urges such as hunger and thirst. The purport is that if one wants, they can pursue separate processes for different types of knowledge, but for one who is devoted to the Lord, the Lord provides all information in the heart as inspiration, after which there is no need for separate endeavors for each type of information. Thus, the meditation on the Paramātma is considered superior to all the other types of practices being performed individually.

Sūtra 3.34
हृदये चत्तिसंवत्
hṛdaye cittasaṁvit

hṛdaye—of the heart; citta—the chitta; saṁvid—complete perception.

TRANSLATION
By the regulatory practice of the heart, complete perception in the chitta.

COMMENTARY
After describing the knowledge and abilities acquired through various types of meditations, the previous sūtra stated that by the talent acquired by spiritual practices everything can be known. And this sūtra states that this talent, which leads to complete perception of everything, is obtained by the regulatory practices of the heart. The regulatory practice of the heart pertains to the devotion to the Lord. A form of the Lord—called Paramātma—resides in the heart. This form pertains to the purposefulness of life. For example, if you are reading a book, then the purpose of the book originally existed in the mind of the author. However, once the book has been produced, then the purpose also exists inside the book. We cannot however perceive this purpose by our senses. This purpose is grasped after we read the book and understand what it is saying. Then we can understand the author's mind, and the intentions underlying the book. The author may also disclose his intentions upfront in the preface or the introduction to the book. In the same way, the Paramātma is the purpose

residing in the heart of every living entity. This purpose is common across all living entities, therefore, the Paramātma is one, even though He exists in the hearts of all living entities. That purpose is the service of the Lord. The Lord also declares this purpose in the scriptures. And if we are interested, the Lord also reveals Himself in the heart. This revelation is recognizing that the purpose of life is devotion to the Lord. Once a soul becomes devoted to the Lord, the Lord provides all guidance from within the heart. The Lord may dictate instructions about how the soul must act, and the soul follows this dictation. As the soul becomes more and more devoted, the Lord also makes His dictation more and more detailed. A pure soul thus speaks the same words as the Lord.

The true yogi devotes himself to the worship of this form in the heart, and by this devotion, the perfection of surrender to the Lord is attained. The Lord then gives the devotee the perfect understanding of everything. Thus, there are many practices by which the yogi can acquire power through their own endeavor. And there is one practice of devotion to the Lord, by which the results of all the other practices are automatically attained by the Lord's grace.

Sūtra 3.35

सत्त्वपुरुषयोरत्यन्तासङ्कीर्णयोःप्रत्ययाविशेषो भोगःपरार्थत्वात्स्वार
थसंयमात्पुरुषज्ञानम्

sattvapuruṣayoratyantāsaṅkīrṇayoḥ pratyayāviśeṣo bhogaḥ
parārthatvātsvārthasaṃyamātpuruṣajñānam

sattva—the truth; puruṣayoh—of the puruṣa; atyanta—extremely; asaṅkīrṇayoḥ—non-complicated; pratyaya—properties and parts; aviśeṣah—without the details; bhogaḥ—enjoyment; para—transcendental; arthatvāt—from being just like purpose; svārtha—self-interest; saṃyamāt—by the regulatory practice; puruṣajñānam—the knowledge of the puruṣa.

TRANSLATION

The truth of the puruṣa is extremely non-complicated; He is transcendental to the enjoyment of the details of the material properties and parts, as if He just has the purpose of being self-interested; the knowledge of the puruṣa is attained by the regulatory practices.

COMMENTARY

The previous sūtra stated that the complete truth is perceived in the heart, and this sūtra elaborates on that truth—He is the puruṣa or the Paramātma. The śrutī describes that there are two souls living in the body—the ātmā and the Paramātma. The ātmā is the individual knower, and the Paramātma is the supreme knower as well as the supreme truth. The Paramātma is self-absorbed, as He is the perfect truth. If the soul becomes absorbed in the understanding of the Paramātma, then he also becomes just like the Paramātma in terms of his experience because both of them are absorbed in the knowledge of the supreme truth. In this regard we can compare the sameness of the experience to empathy. For example, if someone is in emotional pain, and a friend of this person empathizes with this pain, then they can also feel the pain to a great extent. The sameness of the experience doesn't mean the sameness of the personalities. Quite like that, the sameness of the soul's and the Lord's experiences doesn't mean that the soul and the Lord have become identical. But they do become identical in their knowledge and their purpose, without merging their identities. Thus, for all practical purposes, we can say that the soul and the Lord are identical, and yet, they are still separate individuals. This fact is easily understood when we understand the nature of devotion. By devotion, we feel the same as the other person; we know what they know; and we perfectly understand them. In this way, we become almost identical to them, and yet remain distinct.

Some people falsely interpret the puruṣa to be the soul, and they recommend that the soul must become self-absorbed. That self-absorption, however, doesn't give us a complete understanding of reality, because the soul is not the complete reality. The Lord, however, is the complete reality, and by the Lord's assistance in the heart, one can know whatever else needs to be known.

The description of the knowledge of sun, moon, stars, etc. is overridden in this sūtra by stating that the Paramātma is transcendental, the implication being that the other forms of knowledge are not. He is also the complete truth, whereas the others are not the complete truth. Hence, the ultimate goal of yoga is the attainment of the meditation on the Paramātma—the complete truth.

Sūtra 3.36
ततःप्रातभिश्रावणवेदनादर्शास्वादवार्ता जायन्ते
tataḥ prātibhaśravaṇavedanādarśāsvādavārtā jāyante

tataḥ—from that; prātibha—the ability; śravaṇa—hearing; vedanā—touching; darśa—seeing; āsvāda—tasting; vārtā—smelling; jāyante—born inside.

TRANSLATION

From that (concentration in the heart), the ability for (transcendental) hearing, touching, seeing, tasting, and smelling are born inside.

COMMENTARY

The spiritual senses of the soul are meant to glorify the Lord by their activities. When that purpose arises, the desire for glorifying the Lord leads to the creation of the senses. The senses have the capacity to connect to the sense-objects, and thereby understand their nature. However, the abilities of relation and cognition are subordinate to the desire in the senses to enjoy. If the desire doesn't exist, then we don't use the senses. The situation in the material world is somewhat different, because here we are even required to suffer through our senses. Therefore, the material senses exist even if we don't desire to use them. The spiritual senses, however, are manifest for pure pleasure, and that pleasure arises in the relation to the Lord, for the cognition of the Lord, but it can arise only when there is a desire to know the nature of the Lord. Therefore, after preliminary knowledge about the Lord is established in the heart, the soul develops the desire to see the Lord, hear the Lord, touch the Lord, and so on. And the development of these kinds of desires then leads to the spiritual senses.

These spiritual senses are manifest from within the soul, and hence, this body is called the 'internal energy' or antaranga-śakti. The material senses are external to the soul, and act just like the covering of the soul. They are considered not the true senses because they are external. The spiritual senses are instead internal; because they are manifest from within the soul, therefore, they are the true senses. The impersonalist claims that when the material body is destroyed, then the sense perceptions are also destroyed. But this sūtra contradicts such a contention. It says that after realizing that the Paramātma exists in the heart, there is a further development of the spiritual senses. In short, the presence of the Paramātma is realized, and then, through the spiritual senses, the Paramātma is seen, touched, heard, smelt, and even tasted. All these successive sensations are created from hearing itself. Just like we see some food, and the taste buds start watering automatically. Or, we see something beautiful, then the nose also starts feeling a smell. In the same way, when the soul is able to hear the Paramātma in the heart, then gradually he feels all the other sensations. These are the developments of the sensation of hearing the Lord.

Sūtra 3.37
ते समाधावुपसर्गा व्युत्थाने सदिधयः
te samādhāvupasargā vyutthāne siddhayah

te—these (perceptual abilities) samādhau—the samadhi; upasargā—additions; vyutthāne—upon upliftment; siddhayah—are achieved.

TRANSLATION
These perceptual abilities are the additions resulting from the samadhi; they are achieved upon the upliftment (the perfectional state of realization).

COMMENTARY
The senses of the soul are not separate from the soul; they are capacities that exist within the soul, but they are unmanifest, because, for many lifetimes, the soul has forgotten to use its spiritual senses due to reliance on material senses. The soul doesn't realize that it is completely independent of the body, because it has the same capacities as the body, but they are its own capacities. To realize these capacities, the soul must develop the desire to serve the Lord. Hence, when the soul is fully absorbed in the meditation on the Lord, the spiritual senses are automatically manifest due to the development of desire.

In this regard, we must remember that everything is created or manifest for a purpose. The purpose comes first, the functional structure comes next, and the implementation of the functional structure follows. This is true of the material body as well. When the soul enters the material world, it acquires the purpose of sense enjoyment. From that purpose manifests a functional structure in which there are different roles such as seeing, tasting, touching, smelling, hearing, thinking, feeling, willing, judging, intending, and valuing. This functional structure is like the design produced from a purpose. Once this functional design is created, then the design is implemented. And we call that implementation of the design as the body. In the same way, when the soul develops the purpose of loving the Lord, then a functional design of a body suitable for loving the Lord is created. Subsequently, this design is implemented. The functional design is unique to the type of love of the Lord. Thus, for instance, if the soul is interested in loving the Lord as a mother, then a feminine functional structure is created. And from that structure a feminine body is produced.

Since these later steps happen automatically, we should focus not on the type of functional structure or body. We should just focus on developing a strong desire to love the Lord. From that love, everything automatically follows. This process of body creation is identical to that used in the material world.

Sūtra 3.38

बन्धकारणशैथिल्यात्प्रचारसंवेदनाच्च चत्तिस्य परशरीरावेशः

bandhakāraṇaśaithilyātpracārasaṁvedanācca cittasya paraśarīrāveśaḥ

bandhakāraṇa—the cause of bondage; śaithilyāt—upon the weakening; pracāra—progress; saṁvedanā—sensitivity; ca—also; cittasya—of the chitta; paraśarīra—another body; āveśaḥ—possession.

TRANSLATION

Upon the weakening of the cause of bondage, there is the progression of sensitivity (i.e., emotional perceptiveness), also the possession of the chitta in another body (which is capable of acting based on the said emotions).

COMMENTARY

If there is perfect realization of the distinction between the soul and the body, then a practical illustration of this realization is that the soul can enter another body, and the personality of that body would change, because the soul has changed. Sri Shankaracharya is said to have entered the body of a dead king to enjoy sensual pleasures because, during a debate with Mīmāṁsā opponents, he was asked questions about carnal pleasures which he couldn't answer. So, he excused himself from the debate, put his body in the state of samādhī, and entered the body of a king who had just died. He then enjoyed with the king's wives and consorts and obtained a full understanding of sexuality. Then, he left the king's body, returned to his original body, came back to the debate, and defeated his opponents. These abilities are at the soul's disposal if it truly understands the distinction between the soul and the material apparatus, because through this understanding it can attach and detach itself to another body.

Similarly, when the soul develops the desire for serving the Lord, then he also develops the emotional perceptiveness about what the Lord wants, how He feels, and what will make Him happy. The Lord is very shy, and He doesn't truly reveal His innermost desires to everyone. He reveals them only to His devotees, and that revelation follows because the devotees can perceive the Lord's feelings. When the soul begins to understand how the Lord feels, then the Lord also openly reveals His feelings to the devotee. The development of devotion to the Lord gradually leads to the emotional perceptiveness, and by that perceptiveness, the Lord also willingly reveals His nature to the soul.

Sūtra 3.39

उदानजयाज्जलपङ्ककण्टकादिष्वसङ्ग उत्क्रान्तिश्च

udānajayājjalapaṅkakaṇṭakādiṣvasaṅga utkrāntiśca

udāna—the udāna; jayāt—by conquering; jala—water; paṅka—mud; kaṇṭaka—thorns; ādiṣu—etc.; asaṅga—without attachment or contact; utkrānti—passing through; ca—also.

TRANSLATION

By conquering the udāna, one can also pass through water, mud, thorns, etc. without attachment or contact (i.e., without being affected by them).

COMMENTARY

Most people tend to think that if you are far from an object, then you can move toward the object, and this movement involves actions such as walking, running, riding in a car, or a rocket, etc. The real understanding is that the body is fixed although it can interact with other objects, and when it interacts strongly with another object, a sense of proximity to that object is created. This interaction with other objects is indicated in this sūtra through the udāna. By controlling the udāna, anybody can move to any place in the world—even passing through walls, mountains, water, and ground—because factually the body is not moving; the sense of proximity to other things is created through an interaction with them. Thus, if the strength of interaction to the things is increased, then we will find them close to us, and whatever lay in between our body and that object—e.g., walls, mountains, land, water, etc.—would be bypassed. This will give the sense that the person is moving through these things, but factually he is not moving at all. He is just having a sense of proximity to these things, and that proximity can be changed. This is the principle upon which we see various kinds of things in dreams, even though they are not physically close to us. The consciousness of the soul is directed toward certain preexisting realities, and we feel that we are actually seeing them closely. The basis on which we see dreams can also be implemented during waking, by the control of udāna.

Sūtra 3.40

समानजयाज्ज्वलनम्

samānajayājjvalanam

samāna—the samāna; jayāt—by conquering; jvalanam—fire.

TRANSLATION

By conquering the samāna, one can also pass through fire.

COMMENTARY

Modern science claims that proximity to things exerts 'forces' upon us. For example, when we are close to a planet, the planet will exert a force on us. Likewise, if we are close to fire, we will receive more radiation. These claims presuppose a physical sense of proximity, but, as we discussed in the previous sūtra, proximity is itself the byproduct of an interaction. These interactions occur individually for different sense perceptions. For example, it is possible that two things are close for the sense perception of light, but far for the sense perception of heat. Likewise, a thing can be close to earth for the sense perception of light, but far for the sense perception of push and pull. In such cases, we would see that something is passing through fire, but it will not get burnt; or, that something is close to earth, but it is not pulled by the earth's 'gravitational field'. Likewise, as noted in the previous sūtra, we can see someone passing through a wall, but they never feel the resistance of the wall. Or, that they pass through water, but their body never gets wet. The wetness of water, the heat of fire, or the resistance of the wall, are the perceptions of touch, while vision is the perception of sight. At present, we think that all perceptions are equidistant, so if something looks to be close to earth, water, or fire, then it must also be close to receive the sense perception of touch. But this is not always true.

With advancement of scientific understanding, we will see that each sense perception can have a separate distance, due to which all physical theories will become false because they model distance the same way for all properties of an object. For example, quantum mechanics models electrons as particles with the possessed properties of mass and charge, and the distance is accorded to the particle, rather than to the mass and charge. The fact, however, is that mass and charge are separate 'fields' and distance between two masses (which exists in the mass field) can be different from the distance between two charges (which exists in the charge field). If this were to happen, then a physicist will think that the mass or the charge on a particle have reduced (since they are experiencing a reduced force, or no force at all), and then postulate the existence of a particle with that reduced mass or charge. This flawed understanding of distance will lead to infinite such particles as we suppose that if something is close for one sense perception, then it is also close for all other sense perceptions. The real understanding is that the particle and its properties are all fixed, rather than moving, and the appearance of motion is created through an interaction. So, even if the body seems to be inside a wall, it is factually not passing through the wall. It just has an extreme proximity to the wall—for the sense perception of vision. For the sense perception of touch, however, the wall can be far off. So, we might see a yogi passing through a wall, but that yogi may not feel the presence of the wall; others will just see the distance to the wall reduce to zero.

This sūtra, and the previous one, indicate that the sense of proximity between different things is created based on different types of prāṇa. By controlling udāna, we can pass through water without getting wet, and by controlling samāna, without being burnt. Our sense of seeing would therefore indicate that the yogi is passing via fire or water, but his sense of touch will not feel the heat or wetness. A yogi can therefore sit on burning coals and not be burnt by them. Factually, by his control of samāna he has created a distance between the heat of the coal and his sense of touch. So, *we* think that the yogi is sitting on fire, but he is factually not sitting on fire; he is as far as the others seeing him.

Sūtra 3.41
श्रोत्राकाशयोःसम्बन्धसंयमाद्दिव्यं श्रोत्रम्
śrotrākāśayoḥ sambandhasaṁyamāddivyaṁ śrotram

śrotra—the sense of hearing; ākāśayoḥ—the space; sambandha—the relation; saṁyama—by discipline; adi—etc.; divyaṁ—divine; śrotram—hearing.

TRANSLATION
By the discipline of the relation between the sense of hearing and the space, one obtains the capacity for divine hearing.

COMMENTARY
In Sāṅkhya philosophy, matter has five objective properties corresponding to the senses of hearing, touching, seeing, tasting, and smelling. Each of these represent the same meaning, which is perceived by the mind, but to different degrees of elaboration. The sound representation encodes the same meaning (as that which exists in the mind) in the form of a word or sentence. It is a summarized description of the object, which is then further elaborated by the touch, sight, taste, and smell sensations. Therefore, it is not necessary to touch or see an object to know its true nature. We can know that nature simply by hearing. Thus, a yogi can be fully aware of his surroundings, even if his eyes are closed, because he can hear the true nature of things without seeing or touching. We might think that his eyes are closed so he is not seeing the world. But he doesn't have to see or touch. He can also know the surroundings by hearing them.

Sūtra 3.42
कायाकाशयोःसम्बन्धसंयमाल्लघुतूलसमापत्तेश्चाकाशगमनम्
kāyākāśayoḥ
sambandhasaṁyamāllaghutūlasamāpatteścākāśagamanam

kāyā—the body; ākāśayoḥ—the space; sambandha—the relationship;

samyama—regulation; llaghu—light; tūla—cotton; samāpatteh—the wealth; ca—also; ākāśagamanam—movement in the sky.

TRANSLATION

By the discipline of the relation between the body and the space, the wealth of being light just like cotton, and also movement in the sky (is obtained).

COMMENTARY

The so-called gravitational force of modern science is not due to some property called 'mass' that belongs to each object; it is due to the fact that matter is organized in structures, which bind the participating objects into different functional roles. Thus, being part of a structure means being in a certain type of role or relationship to other things. Our place or role in a system is determined by our karma, and, due to karma, we belong to some society, some family, some organization, and some planet. Hence, our body is 'tied' to earth due to our karma, not due to gravity. When the constrains of karma are transcended, then the body can freely move in space without a rocket or spaceship. This movement occurs by using the preexisting karma to enter new relationships.

Karma is just like money; we can use it in different ways. So, if a yogi has accumulated good karma, then he can enter other planets. The process for this entry is the same—through our prāṇa we establish proximity to another reality, and then we are immediately transported into another world. Our power of creating proximity, however, will work only if we have the requisite karma. Hence, the yogis perform great austerities to accumulate good karma, and realize the power of prāṇa to create proximity. Then, by the combination of the power, and their good karma, they transport themselves to other planets. Even if they did not transport themselves in this way, the laws of karma will automatically transport them to other planets at the time of death. The difference is simply that the yogi—if he transfers himself—will go to the new planet in the same body. But if the laws of karma transfer the yogi, then a new body would be required. In the former case, the body is moving to a new place, and in the latter case, the soul is moving across different bodies. The net result of these two mechanisms is the same, and this means that the yogi can retain his body and yet experience alternative places and lifestyles in the same type of body.

Sūtra 3.43

वहरिकल्पतिा वृत्तरिमहावदिेहा ततःप्रकाशावरणक्षयः

vahirakalpitā vṛttirmahāvidehā tataḥ prakāśāvaraṇakṣayaḥ

vahir—carrying; akalpitā—unimaginable; vṛttir—capacities; mahā—great; videhā—without a body; tataḥ—thereafter; prakāśa—light or conscious experience; āvaraṇa—the covering; kṣayaḥ—the destruction of.

TRANSLATION

Carrying unimaginable capacities, the great soul lives without a body; thereafter, the covering of conscious experience is also destroyed.

COMMENTARY

The material body, senses, mind, intellect, ego, and the moral sense are various coverings of the soul that need to exist only if we desire and deserve a certain type of experience. As the soul is purified of the various kinds of desiring and deserving, those bodies are also destroyed. We can compare this to a person removing the various layers of clothing one after another. Just as at the time of death the gross body is left behind, and the soul moves to another gross body, similarly, the soul can leave behind the bodies of senses, mind, intellect, ego, and the moral sense, and exist in the subtle body of guna, karma, and chitta. If the yogi has no bad karma, then he is not forced to suffer. He can keep his consciousness withdrawn, and ultimately discard even the subtle body.

Sūtra 3.44

स्थूलस्वरूपसूक्ष्मान्वयार्थवत्त्वसंयमादभूतजयः

sthūlasvarūpasūkṣmānvayārthavattvasaṁyamādbhūtajayaḥ

sthūla—gross; svarūpa—the form; sūkṣma—subtle; anvaya—different; arthavattva—as if meaning; samyama—regulation; adbhūta—the gross material elements; jayaḥ—victory.

TRANSLATION

Their gross and subtle forms are the different forms of meaning; these forms give complete control over the gross elements, and victory (over them).

COMMENTARY

The terms 'gross' and 'subtle' do not have an absolute meaning. Even the term 'chitta' doesn't have a fixed meaning. As we have discussed, the chitta is the abilities of cognition and conation using which the soul tries to acquire greatness in this world. A crude sense of greatness is that a person owns a lot of wealth. A more subtle sense of greatness is that he understands the working of the mind and the senses and is able to control them. An even more subtle greatness is the possession of mystical powers. And a further subtle greatness is liberation from the material entanglement. Ultimately, the subtlest sense of greatness is devotion to the Lord. Thus, as the ideas of greatness change, the abilities in the chitta adapt accordingly, and the gross body also changes.

As the conceptions of greatness become more subtle, one obtains greater mastery over the gross reality. Spiritual elevation means rising up this inverted tree from the gross to the subtle. And with this rising, there is natural capacity to control what lies lower in this tree. Thus, even if a yogi has subtle and gross bodies, these are not like our bodies, because the definition of 'gross' and 'subtle' is relative to the idea of greatness; if our ideas of greatness become subtle, then, the gross body also becomes subtler. Hence, this sūtra says that the gross and subtle bodies of the yogis are not like our body; they are forms of meaning. Of course, even our bodies are forms of meaning. But the yogi's body is even subtler meanings. And with their senses and mind they can easily control all other bodies that are relatively grosser. Just like a fine instrument can measure large things, but a large instrument cannot measure fine things, similarly, a subtle body can control the gross body, and thus the yogi obtains great powers.

Sūtra 3.45
ततोऽणिमादिप्रादुर्भावःकायसम्पत्तद्धर्मानभिघातश्च
tato'ṇimādiprādurbhāvaḥ kāyasampattaddharmānabhighātaśca

tatah—from that; aṇimādi—the mystical power of anima etc.; prādurbhāvaḥ—are born; kaya—body; sampattad—the wealth; dharma—duty and religiosity; anabhighāta—never hurt or injured; ca—also.

TRANSLATION

From that (powerful body) the mystical powers of animā etc. are born; with the wealth of such body, the duty and religiosity are also never compromised.

COMMENTARY

Most people imagine that if they had yogic powers, then they would be able to use them to obtain great mastery over the world. But this sūtra states that by the time someone acquires such powers, their desire to exploit material nature for selfish ends disappears. These powers are not easily obtained, but if they have been obtained, the person knows the risks in misusing them. If they are misused, the result is much greater bad karma because the effects of misuse are also much greater. Thus, the person with such mystical powers only uses them for performing his duties, and never for any personal aggrandizement. There are eight such mystical powers, called anima, laghima, mahima, garima, etc.

Anima: the ability to shrink one's body size to that of an atom. An example is Hanuman reducing his size while searching for Sita.

Mahima: the ability to become as large as one wants. Hanuman display this mystic power while setting Lanka on fire.

Garima: the ability to become heavier. Hanuman made his tail so heavy that even the very powerful Bhima couldn't lift it.

Laghima: the ability to make one's body weightless and fly in the air. Hanuman displayed this mystic power when he flew to Lanka.

Prapti: the ability to obtain anything anywhere. This means that one is able to reduce the distance to anything at will.

Prakamya: this enables the power to live in any environment, such as water, fire, enter the body of another person, etc.

Isitva: the power to ascend to any position of rulership. By this power, one can control societies and planets, and control other living entities.

Vasitva: this is the ability to bring other people's minds and senses under their control, and make them think or do as you desire.

Sūtra 3.46

रूपलावण्यबलवज्रसंहननत्वानि कायसम्पत्

rūpalāvaṇyabalavajrasaṁhananatvāni kāyasampat

rūpa—form; lāvaṇya—beauty; bala—power; vajrasaṁ—hard like vajra; hananatvāni—in destroying; kāyasampat—the wealth of the body.

TRANSLATION

The wealth of the yogi's body includes a beautiful form, power, and hard like vajra in destroying.

COMMENTARY

We might think that the practice of spiritual life requires the rejection of material enjoyment, and that is true to an extent. However, more important than the superficial rejection of such enjoyment is the desire for such pleasure. Because as one accumulates mystical powers, and the desires for material enjoyment are intact, these powers are used for the same kinds of pleasures as ordinary people. This sūtra notes how the yogi can attain a beautiful body, that is extremely powerful. One might wonder: Why would anyone undergo such hardship to attain the same results as may be obtained by other means? But if the material desires are not destroyed, then such results of yoga are possible.

Sūtra 3.47

ग्रहणस्वरूपास्मितान्वयार्थवत्त्वसंयमादिन्द्रियजयः

grahaṇasvarūpāsmitānvayārthavattvasaṁyamādindriyajayaḥ

grahaṇa—the acceptance; svarūpa—the form; asmitā—ego or pride; anvayārthavattva—just as for other purposes; saṁyamādi—by regulation; indriyajayaḥ—the conquest of the senses.

TRANSLATION

On the acceptance of such a form, there is ego or pride just as for the other purposes (of sense enjoyment); by regulation, one must conquer the senses.

COMMENTARY

This sūtra warns the potential seeker of mystical powers of the dangers of acquiring them. Naturally with such immense power, there is a possibility of egotism which can lead a person to misusing the power. That misuse will then lead to the yogi's fall. Hence, this sūtra states that the yogi must control his senses by regulation, and not allow himself to be misled by his great powers. If used for dharma, the powers are a great boon. But the same powers can also be used for adharma and that misuse would then destroy the yogi's powers.

Sūtra 3.48
ततो मनोजवित्वं विकिरणभावःप्रधानजयश्च
tato manojavitvaṁ vikaraṇabhāvaḥ pradhānajayaśca

tato—from that (regulation of the senses despite immense powers); mano—the mind; javitvaṁ—swiftness; vikaraṇa—different or orthogonal; bhāvaḥ—nature; pradhāna—the pradhāna; jayaśca—also conquers.

TRANSLATION
From that (regulation of the senses despite immense powers) the mind becomes swift; acquiring a different nature, it also conquers pradhāna.

COMMENTARY
Our minds can receive or transmit information from only one source at a time, not from or to simultaneous sources at the same time. Likewise, the rate at which they can receive or transmit information is also finite. The process of reception of information is called prāṇa. Once this information is received, it must be reformulated according to our understanding, and that process is called samāna or 'digestion' of information. Once the information is digested, then it must be given a proper place, and this is called vyāna or 'circulation' of information. As a result of new information, some old information may be discarded, and this process is called apāna. Finally, we might seek a certain type of information and move toward it, which is called udāna. For material information, generally all five of these processes are involved, and this process of moving, absorbing, digesting, assimilating, and discarding ideas is slow.

However, when a person becomes spiritually realized, then there is no need for discarding information, digesting information, or rearranging information, because everything is seen just as it is. Then, the conventional knowledge acquisition seems too slow, because it involves acquiring, digesting, assimilating, and moving the ideas before an action is taken. As a yogi becomes advanced, all these processes occur very rapidly, and therefore a person with such advancement is able to act very fast compared to the other people. Even in this world we can see some people are very quick in grasping the essence of things, while others take a long time to understand them. Some people are able to act very fast, while others are very slow. Factually, the mind is very powerful and as one advances spiritually, the mind becomes extremely agile—it is able to assimilate, understand, transform, and abandon the ideas very quickly.

Other people may find this quite surprising, as they generally struggle to do simple things. But these things are not surprising to the advanced soul. This sūtra states that with yogic advancement, the mind becomes so fast that it can understand everything quickly. At that point, the yogi may lose interest in interacting with the dull and sluggish people; he may desire to associate only with those who are as good as he is. By this desire of associating with others who are as intelligent as he is, the yogi loses all interest in the people who are ignorant. Of course, a devotee of the Lord remains humble and tries to elevate others even if the process seems very hard. But the yogi who is not such a devotee, completely loses interest in ordinary people. Thus, he transcends the pradhāna, because whatever seems great to ordinary people seems ordinary to the yogi. By his desire to seek something even greater, he rejects the material greatness.

Sūtra 3.49

सत्त्वपुरुषान्यताख्यातिमात्रस्य सर्वभावाधिष्ठातृत्वं सर्वज्ञातृत्वं च

sattvapuruṣānyatākhyātimātrasya
sarvabhāvādhiṣṭhātṛtvaṁ sarvajñātṛtvaṁ ca

sattva—the mode of pure goodness; puruṣa—the Lord; anyatā—otherness; khyātimātrasya—only for name-sake; sarvabhāvādhiṣṭhātṛtvaṁ—as the master of all existence; sarvajñātṛtvaṁ—as the knower of everything; ca—also.

TRANSLATION

In that mode of pure goodness (i.e., without tamo-guna and rajo-guna), anything other the Lord is only for name-sake; He is seen as the master of all existence, and as the knower of everything as well.

COMMENTARY

The Lord cannot be understood by our material minds and senses, because He is the source of everything, the controller of everything, and the knower of everything. Knowing Him means knowing everything. We cannot understand the nature of everything with our material mind and senses. For that, we need senses and a mind that are not constrained by the material nature, as noted in the previous sūtra. Once we see the Lord, and understand that He is the source of everything, then we realize that there is nothing other than the Lord. Even the soul is understood as being a part of the Lord. Therefore, our knowing the Lord is a part of the Lord knowing the whole. And because this whole is the source of everything, therefore, it has contradictory qualities. As long as we are ourselves situated in the contradictory modes of rajo-guna and tamo-guna, we can understand one side of this contradiction, but when we switch to the other side, we will forget the previous side, or find that it doesn't exist. Therefore, to know the whole truth, we must be free of the material conditioning. What is that freedom? It means that there something that is without the tradeoffs of material nature where increase in one quality means a decrease in the opposite quality. If one transcends this condition of thinking in terms of opposites, then he can understand the true nature of reality as it is beyond the opposites.

The previous sūtra stated that the yogi transcends pradhāna, which is the mundane ideas of greatness. What is this greatness? It is the attraction to ordinary pleasures of life. For example, natural beauty seems great to ordinary people. Some people are attracted to wealth and power. They see people holding high positions and they imagine themselves having a similar kind of power. The true yogi however transcends all these notions of greatness, as they become boring for him. He rather seeks true greatness, which is devoid of the limitations of this world. This greatness is found in the Lord. So, the true yogi seeks shelter in the knowledge of the Lord, as the world has become too boring.

Sūtra 3.50
तद्वैराग्यादपि दोषवीजक्षये कैवल्यम्
tadvairāgyādapi doṣavījakṣaye kaivalyam

tadvairāgyād—after detachment from material nature; api—even; doṣavījakṣaye—the seed of faults is destroyed; kaivalyam—liberation.

TRANSLATION

After detachment from material nature, even the seeds of faults are destroyed, leading to liberation.

COMMENTARY

The impersonalist believes that liberation is different from the perfect knowledge of the Lord, and this sūtra refutes this. It states that when one is completely detached from material opposites, and the Lord is experienced as the whole truth, then there is automatic liberation. The reason is that even if we reject the material dualities, we cannot stay permanently in that state, because it is devoid of all experience. For the liberation to be permanent, we must know that truth which is both of the opposites, and yet, neither of the material opposites. Therefore, complete knowledge of the Lord is identical to liberation, and whatever is considered 'liberation' merely due to the detachment of the material modes is temporary. Thus, if someone wants the liberation to be permanent, then they should try to understand the nature of the Supreme Lord, because by that knowledge, the detachment and liberation are automatically obtained.

Sūtra 3.51

स्थान्युपनिमन्त्रणे सङ्गस्मयाकरणं पुनरनिष्टप्रसङ्गात्

sthānyupanimantraṇe saṅgasmayākaraṇaṁ punaraniṣṭaprasaṅgāt

sthānya—the place; upanimantraṇe—upon the invitation; saṅgasmaya—desiring the association; ākaraṇaṁ—do not do that; punar—again; aniṣṭaprasaṅgāt—from the incidence of undesirable results.

TRANSLATION

Upon the invitation to ascend a higher position, one should not accept that position, desiring the association (of a powerful position), as it again leads to undesirable results.

COMMENTARY

As a transcendentalist advances in spiritual life, he is offered various kinds of material allurements such as power, wealth, superior position of leadership, respect and recognition, and heavenly sexual pleasure. The material nature gives the soul a vision of various kinds of enjoyments to tempt him away from his transcendental pursuits, and many yogis fall prey to that attraction. This sūtra says that when they do that, over time they lose the position and power, and they fall again into the same condition as before. Everything in material nature declines. Even our memory declines over time. As we become allured by material enjoyments, we forget the transcendental purpose. And then, as time passes, even the extraordinary mystical powers are lost, because they are just like the abilities of our hands and legs to lift heavy things or run. Aging in this world makes our hands and legs weak. Similarly, aging in the heavenly planets makes the mystical powers of the residents there weak. As they lose their mystical abilities, they fall again into the ordinary life forms, where they have better capacities than ordinary mortals, and can enjoy greater power, wealth, fame, and resources for some more time. But time destroys everything, and with its passing, the yogi descends to the condition of all other beings. The intelligent yogi therefore realizes that ascending to a position of greater power is a trap for temporary enjoyment, that eventually descends into ignominy.

Sūtra 3.52
क्षणतत्क्रमयोःसंयमाद्वविकजं ज्ञानम्
kṣaṇatatkramayoḥ saṁyamādvivekajaṁ jñānam

kṣaṇa—momentary; tat—that; kramayoḥ—sequence; saṁyamād—by regulation; vivekajaṁ—intelligence is born; jñānam—leading to knowledge.

TRANSLATION
Momentary is that sequence (of ascending and descending); by regulation intelligence is born, which leads to the true knowledge.

COMMENTARY
Here a clear distinction is drawn between the momentary pleasures of heavenly planets and the eternal happiness of the spiritual realization. If one is allured by temporary pleasures, then he loses the prospect of eternal happiness. Therefore, the yogi is advised—don't be tempted by these things; regulate your mind and focus on the true goal of life, rather than

the temporary distractions. The principle of detachment thus holds true not just in the preliminary stages of life. It rather holds true even for the advancing yogi. In fact, as the yogi advances, ever more alluring temptations are presented. The material nature thus tests the conviction of the yogi, and those who fail that test repeat the cycle of birth and death. Those who pass this test, however, surpass this world.

Sūtra 3.53
जातिलक्षणदेशैरन्यतानवच्छेदात्तुल्ययोस्ततःप्रतिपत्तिः
jātilakṣaṇadeśairanyatānavacchedāttulyayostataḥ pratipattiḥ

jāti—class; lakṣaṇa—symptoms; deśa—place; iranyata—and other ways; anavacchedāt—due to the undivided; tulyayostataḥ—not comparable to that; pratipattiḥ—the surrender to the Lord.

TRANSLATION
The surrender to the Lord (leads to a place), which is undivided (by dualities), and cannot be compared in class, symptoms, place, or any other way (to the mundane world).

COMMENTARY
Once the attainments of ordinary material world are rejected, the glories of the Supreme Lord's abode are described. The abodes of this material world are dualistic; for example, you cannot get something that is simultaneously hard and soft, rough and smooth, great and humble, beautiful and tough, etc. All these qualities are separated from each other and this separation constitutes the notion of material space. The spiritual space, on the other hand, is constituted of non-duality, in which the opposites coexist simultaneously. The Supreme Lord has all qualities, and things close to Him are almost like Him. As one moves farther away from the Supreme Lord, fewer qualities are seen, but even then, opposites are simultaneously present. Only when the soul falls into the material world, that the opposites become exclusive. Thus, in this world, we are accustomed to a materialistic logic in which the presence of one quality must mean the absence of its opposite. Thus, the source of the spiritual space is 'everything', and the source of material space is 'nothing'. When something originates from 'everything' it carries the opposing qualities of everything. But

when something originates from 'nothing', then it carries one of the many opposing qualities, and none of the places in this world can be compared to the spiritual world as all the material places are missing something, and due to that incompleteness, nobody can be totally satisfied in that place. As one tries to overcome this incompleteness, he imbibes a new quality, but loses the previous quality, and this causes a cyclical change in this world. The spiritual world is however eternal because those places do not experience any kind of incompleteness.

Sūtra 3.54

तारकं सर्ववषियं सर्वथावषियमक्रमं चेति विवेकजं ज्ञानम्

tārakaṁ sarvaviṣayaṁ sarvathāviṣayamakramaṁ ceti vivekajaṁ jñānam

tārakaṁ—upon transcendence; sarvaviṣayaṁ—all the subjects; sarvathā—at all times; viṣayam—enjoyed; akramaṁ—without sequence; ca—also; iti—in this way; vivekajaṁ—true intellect; jñānam—is called knowledge.

TRANSLATION

Upon transcendence, all the subjects are enjoyed at all the times, without sequencing; in this way also, the true intellect is called knowledge.

COMMENTARY

As already noted, the material world is defined by dualities. If you are enjoying working, then you cannot enjoy sleeping. If you are enjoying eating, then you cannot enjoy running. If you are seeing one thing, then you cannot see other things. And if one type of belief is held, then the opposite belief must be rejected. The senses of hearing, touching, seeing, tasting, and smelling operate one after another. When consciousness is focused on thought, then sensation is ignored. When we are focused on enjoyment, we forget our duties, but when we are performing our duties, we must sacrifice our enjoyment. In this way, the material world is 'sequenced' from one quality to another. This sūtra states that the spiritual world is 'not sequenced', and everything can be enjoyed at all times. This type of cognition, relation, and emotion is called true knowledge.

Sūtra 3.55
सत्त्वपुरुषयोःशुद्धिसाम्ये कैवल्यमिति
sattvapuruṣayoḥ śuddhisāmye kaivalyamiti

sattva—the essence; puruṣayoḥ—of the Supreme Lord; śuddhi—purity; sāmye—similarity to; kaivalyamiti—is known as liberation.

TRANSLATION

The essence that is similar to the purity of the Supreme Lord is liberation.

COMMENTARY

The Supreme Lord is perfection, and that means that when He possesses one quality, it doesn't mean that He doesn't possess the opposite quality. Thus, He is soft toward His devotees, and hard toward the demonic. He is deeply attached to those who love Him, and He is unattached to those who ignore Him. He looks beautiful to those who appreciate Him, and He looks ferocious to those who criticize Him. He is weak and compliant in the face of love, and He is strong and resilient in the face of opponents. He craves attention from those who cannot live without Him, and He remains indifferent to those who don't care about Him. He is everything, but He manifests the quality which we desire to see. As we relate to the Supreme Lord, He relates the same way to us.

The perfected soul has the same qualities as the Lord. He can be arrogant toward the arrogant, and humble toward the humble. He can be kind to those who are kind, and harsh toward those who are harsh. He acts like a fool before the intelligent, but he acts intelligent toward the fools. He is attached to those who are attached to the Lord, and he ignores those who are envious of the Lord. Thus, it is impossible to categorize or classify the devotee of the Lord by mundane qualities, because he is not universally humble or arrogant, kind or harsh, fool or intelligent, attached or unattached. He is everything, but he manifests that aspect of his personality which is required and needed in a situation.

In this way, the devotee of the Lord is just like the Lord—namely, that he possesses opposite qualities. Ordinary people see these opposites in him and are confused. They might argue: You said this earlier, and today you are saying something different. This is because they are accustomed to a mundane universalizing tendency in which a person must always be categorized in the same way. The pure soul, however, cannot be categorized because he is just like the Lord. Therefore, the scriptures state that the ordinary people should not try to imitate the devotees; they should rather just follow the instructions of that person. The pure devotee might impart different instructions to different people, in different times, and places. This is for their own good. But those who try to universalize these instructions don't understand how the Lord is everything in a universal sense, but is something different in each time, place, and situation. The devotee also is different in each time, place, and situation. Thus, the most common attribute of advanced devotees is that they are totally unpredictable.

CHAPTER 4

Sūtra 4.1
जन्मौषधिमन्त्रतपःसमाधिजाःसिद्धियः
janmauṣadhimantratapaḥsamādhijāḥ siddhayaḥ

janma—birth; auṣadhi—medicine; mantra—the divine sounds; tapaḥ—austerity; samādhijāḥ—giving birth to samadhi; siddhayaḥ—on perfection.

TRANSLATION
The medicines for birth are the divine sounds and austerities; they give rise to Samādhī on perfection.

COMMENTARY
Birth and death are considered illnesses in yoga philosophy. They are not the normal state of existence of the soul, which is eternal. The cure for this illness is the chanting of mantras and the performance of austerities. When these practices are followed, then the soul becomes the same as the origin—i.e., the Lord—and overcomes the cycle of repeated birth and death. Samādhī means full absorption and austerities are the means for detachment. Therefore, a two-pronged approach is recommended to become detached from the material life and become attached to the Lord. Those who practice detachment from matter but don't get attached to the Lord fall again into the material world. And those who practice attachment to the Lord, but don't get detached from the material world, keep rowing a boat of spiritual advancement that is tied to the shore. Hence, both attachment and detachment are recommended simultaneously.

Sūtra 4.2
जात्यन्तरपरिणामःप्रकृत्यापूरात्
jātyantarapariṇāmaḥ prakṛtyāpūrāt

jāti—the species; antara—differences; pariṇāmaḥ—the results; prakṛti—the material nature; āpūrāt—due to fulfilling the desires.

TRANSLATION

The results of the different species are due to prakṛti fulfilling the desires.

COMMENTARY

Each species of life is ideally suited for the fulfilment of a different kind of desire. The tiger body is well-suited for hunting, the birds are well-suited for flying, and the fishes are well-suited for swimming. Each species of life consumes a different kind of food, builds a different kind of shelter, enjoys sex in a different way, and rears children in a different way. Thus, the different species of life exist not due to genetic mutations, but because there are different kinds of desires and inclinations, and the material diversity exists to fulfill them.

Sūtra 4.3

नमित्तिमप्रयोजकं प्रकृतीनां वरणभेदस्तु ततःक्षेत्रकिवत्

nimittamaprayojakaṁ prakṛtīnāṁ varaṇabhedastu tataḥ kṣetrikavat

nimittam—the purpose; aprayojakaṁ—not instigating or prompting; prakṛtīnām—due to prakṛti; varaṇa—selecting or choosing; bhedastu—only due to differences; tataḥ—in those; kṣetrikavat—just like the fields.

TRANSLATION

The purpose (of enjoyment) is not due to prakṛti instigating or prompting them; they are only due to the differences in the selection in those (living entities) just like the selection of different fields (for growing different crops).

COMMENTARY

The impersonalist attributes the material entanglement to material nature, saying that nature deludes the soul into enjoyment. This sūtra refutes that conclusion. In the Sāṅkhya Sūtra, it is stated that the only purpose of material nature is to purify the soul of its material desires. But if the soul harbors such desires, material nature facilitates its enjoyment.

This sūtra states the same conclusion in a different way: It describes the various species of life just like different fields in to which the farmer plants different kinds of seeds. This is a common theme across all Vedic texts in which the soul is held responsible for its entanglement and liberation; the entanglement is due to the soul's desires to become the lord and master, and liberation is obtained when this desire for being the lord and master is discarded, and the soul surrenders to the Lord and becomes His servant. The Lord and material nature are not responsible or accountable for the soul's enjoyment or suffering; they merely facilitate it.

Sūtra 4.4
नर्मिाणचति्तान्यस्मितामात्रात्
nirmāṇacittānyasmitāmātrāt

nirmāṇa—construction; cittāni—the chitta; asmitāmātrāt—from only due to the egotism.

TRANSLATION
(The various species) are constructed from the chitta only due to egotism.

COMMENTARY
As we have discussed, the pradhāna is the idea that I am the lord, master, controller, and enjoyer. The chitta is manifest from pradhāna as the collection of previously acquired abilities. The root of the problem, however, lies in the soul's egotism where it wants to become independent of the Lord and accepts the ideas of lordship, mastery, controllership, and enjoyment as the proofs or evidence of that independence. Thus, each soul in the material world is similar in the sense that everyone is trying to become great. They are however different in the type of greatness they have chosen for themselves. This variety in the types of greatness is a material creation. However, the root idea of trying to be great—or trying to imitated the Lord—is the egotism within the soul.

Sūtra 4.5
प्रवृत्तभिेदे प्रयोजकं चति्तमेकमनेकेषाम्
pravṛttibhede prayojakaṁ cittamekamanekeṣām

pravṛttibhede—the variations in tendencies; prayojakaṁ—engagement or experimentation; cittam—the chitta; ekam—one; anekeṣām—into many.

TRANSLATION

Due to the variations in tendencies, one chitta manifests into many types of engagements or experimentation.

COMMENTARY

As we have discussed, from the skills and the abilities in the chitta manifest the desires for a specific kind of mastery, from the desires of mastery manifest the ideas about greatness, and from the ideas of greatness manifests the ego. These are the modifications of the chitta, just like the waves in an ocean. If someone believes that greatness is power and wealth, then he sometimes pursues power to acquire wealth, and sometimes wealth to acquire power. If the notion of power dominates, then one tries to steal other people's wealth. But if the notion of wealth dominates, then he tries to control the rulers of a country by wealth. Thus, many varieties of mastery are created by the divisions and combinations of the primitive ideas of greatness. The problem is that if you get one type of greatness, then you lose another type of greatness. Thus, the rich people are forced to part with their wealth due to taxes, and they give away wealth to politicians to reduce this loss. Similarly, even though the politician is supposed to be strong, he becomes a slave to the rich, because his power alone is not enough. In this way, there is constant struggle to become great, and one type of lordship is traded for another, but the soul is never completely satisfied.

Sūtra 4.6

तत्र ध्यानजमनाशयम्
tatra dhyānajamanāśayam

tatra—there; dhyāna—by meditation; jama—is born; nāśayam—the destruction.

TRANSLATION

In that chitta, by meditation is born the destruction (of the tendencies).

COMMENTARY

The ideas of the self being the lord and master of the world, and the resulting attempts to prove this lordship and mastery over the world are all false. If the soul performs some good deeds, then he gets some lordship and mastery temporarily. And when he acquires this power, he inevitably misuses it. After all, what kind of lordship would it be if the soul could not do whatever he wanted? The soul's delusion of its mastery thus leads to its fall from power, because when the power is misused, bad karma is created. Thus, a cycle of good and bad deeds leads to a cycle of rise and fall. If, however, the soul meditates on the Lord, then he realizes that he is not the lord and master of the world. The Lord is the true controller. His greatness is unsurpassed, and the soul can never displace the Lord as the lord and master of the world. That meditation then destroys the false ideas of greatness, and thereby of the experiments to prove the mastery. Now, the soul accepts the Lord's pleasure as his life's purpose. And this frees the soul from the cycle of birth and death as the truth is now known, and the delusionary attempts at greatness are totally terminated.

Sūtra 4.7
कर्माशुक्लाकृष्णं योगिनस्त्रिविधमितरेषाम्
karmāśuklākṛṣṇaṁ yoginastrividhamitareṣām

karma—the actions; aśukla—not white; akṛṣṇaṁ—not black; yoginah—of the yogis; trividham—three-fold; itareṣām—of the others.

TRANSLATION

The actions of the yogis are not black or white; of others they are three-fold.

COMMENTARY

The actions are classified in three ways—(1) those leading to good results, (2) those leading to bad results, (3) those leading to no result. These are respectively called sukarma, vikarma, and akarma. If someone thinks that the actions of the yogis are just like those of the others—i.e., good, and bad—then this sūtra refutes this contention. It states that the actions of the yogis are neither good nor bad—neither white nor black. Then, these actions must be classified into the third category—namely, akarma, or those which have no consequences.

Karma is not difficult to understand. When a person is employed in a job, his actions produce some effects—which are called 'work'. Then, at the end of the month, he is paid some salary—which is called his 'compensation'. Thus, there is one action—the work—and there are two results— (1) the effects, and (2) the consequences. Karma is, similarly, like the consequences of actions. The difference is simply that compensation is only of one type (i.e., that the employee is paid at the end of the month) but karma is of three kinds (good, bad, and neither). The neither category of consequences is produced if our duties are performed without the expectation of results. This can happen in multiple ways. For example, someone can perform duty for the sake of being dutiful, and not expect a recompense in return; this is called karma-yoga. Likewise, one can perform their duty due to devotion to the Lord, expecting not a material reward, but the pleasure of the Lord; this process is called bhakti-yoga. Thus, the yogi's actions, if they are performed either without a desire for any result, or due to the desire for the Lord's pleasure (which is a spiritual, not a material desire), are classified as akarma. All other actions create good or bad karma.

Sūtra 4.8

ततस्तद्वपिाकानुगुणानामेवाभिव्यक्तिर्वासनानाम्

tatastadvipākānuguṇānāmevābhivyaktirvāsanānām

tatastad—from those (three kinds of results); vipāka—the adverse results; anuguṇānām—according to one's nature or qualities; eva—certainly; abhivyaktih—are expressed due to; vāsanānām—the materialistic desires.

TRANSLATION

From those (three kinds of results), the adverse results are certainly manifest due to the materialistic desires, according to one's nature or qualities.

COMMENTARY

In the law of karma, enjoyments are optional, but suffering is mandatory—as long as we are not free of material desires. Since the enjoyments are optional, therefore, a person with good karma can renounce materialistic pleasures and lead a simple life, or even perform severe austerities. Enjoyments are delivered due to good karma to a person only when he desires it. However, nobody desires suffering, and yet, it comes anyway. As long as we have any material desires, their very opposite would be delivered to us as suffering. Thus, a lazy person is punished by making him work hard. And a hard-working person is punished by depriving him of work. A sociable person is punished by isolating them, and a loner is punished by forcing community on them. In this way, karma acts in the just the opposite way to our desires. But if all material desires are destroyed, then karma is also destroyed because there is nothing likable, so there is nothing dislikable. Without some liking and disliking, how can there be enjoyment and suffering? Therefore, this sūtra states that as long as there are materialistic desires, suffering is also mandatory according to our nature.

Sūtra 4.9

जातदिशकालव्यवहितानामप्यानन्तर्यं स्मृतसिंस्कारयोरेकरूपत्वात्

jātideśakālavyavahitānāmapyānantaryaṁ
smṛtisaṁskārayorekarūpatvāt

jāti—species; deśa—place; kāla—time; vyavahitānāma—separated; api—even; ānantaryaṁ—proximity; smṛti—the memory; saṁskārayoh—the impressions from the past; ekarūpatvāt—due to as if having the same form.

TRANSLATION

Even though the species are separated by place and time, due to proximity with the memory of past impressions, they seem as if having the same form.

COMMENTARY

In modern time, most people think of the various species in terms of their bodily shape and size, and they believe that the mind is a byproduct of this gross bodily form. This sūtra however states that the gross bodily form arises due to the impressions of the chitta. And these impressions are called 'memory' because they are carried over from one life and body to another. Thus, for instance, humans are present all over the world, but there are some core values—such as an interest in what lies beyond our current existence—that define the human nature. Humans have a curiosity about nature, they want to know how things work, and how they came about. This curiosity is absent in animals. Similarly, different animal species have a likeness with each other, and these manifest in two other things besides the bodily shape and form: (1) their behaviors, and (2) their purposes. A species is not defined merely by the shape and size of the body, but also by their behaviors (which we can see), and by how they feel, what goals they have, what they like or dislike, etc. (which we cannot see). Modern science is based on the third-person perspective about species, but their behaviors can be explained only if we see how these bodies have social relations, which constitute the second-person perspective. Similarly, the emotions and purposes felt by each member of the species are the first-person perspective. When we broaden our definition of 'species' then we obtain a more complete understanding of what it means to belong to a particular class of life forms.

Sūtra 4.10

तासामनादित्वं चाशिषो नित्यत्वात्

tāsāmanāditvaṁ cāśiṣo nityatvāt

tāsām—from these; anāditvaṁ—without beginning; ca—also; āśiṣo—the blessings (i.e., their byproducts); nityatvāt—due to as if eternal.

TRANSLATION

From these beginningless impressions, also, the blessings (i.e., their byproducts) are produced due to as if they were eternal.

COMMENTARY

Modern psychology recognizes that the unconscious is far bigger than the conscious memories, but it doesn't dive into why that unconscious is bigger. If we have only lived this particular life, then all the memories must only be comprised of what we have experienced in this life. We might not remember some of these, but we remember a lot of it. If that is indeed the case, then the unconscious must be comparable to the conscious. For a person who has good memory, their unconscious must be smaller than the conscious. And that would also mean that our thoughts must be constrained by what we have seen in this life. Genuinely new ideas thus cannot appear, and this means that radical scientific theories, or inventions about what has not been seen, are impossible. Similarly, a person cannot be born with innate tendencies toward art, music, poetry, or sports, as they don't have sufficient encounter with these things. Since we cannot explain these occurrences, therefore, we must accept that the unconscious is formed in earlier lives but carried from one body to another.

Sūtra 4.11
हेतुफलाश्रयालम्बनैःसङ्गृहीतत्वादेषामभावे तदभावः
hetuphalāśrayālambanaiḥ saṅgṛhītatvādeṣāmabhāve tadabhāvaḥ

hetu—the purpose; phala—the results; āśraya—the shelter; ālambanaiḥ—taking support of; saṅgṛhītatvāt—due to being accumulated; eṣām—these; abhāve—in the absence of; tadabhāvaḥ—that (body) is also absent.

TRANSLATION
Taking the shelter and support of the accumulated purpose and the results, in the absence of these (impressions) leads to the absence of that (body).

COMMENTARY
As we have discussed, the unconscious comprises of three parts—the chitta, guna, and karma. The chitta has been discussed in the last sūtra, and this sūtra refers to the guna (the purpose) and karma (the results). It is not enough to just have impressions; we must also *like* the thoughts arising in us, and we must get the *opportunity* to fulfill these likes. The liking and disliking are called guna, and the opportunities to fulfill these likes and dislikes is called karma. Hence, this sūtra says that the thoughts arising out of the chitta take shelter and support of the purpose and the results. The term 'shelter' refers to the guna, and the term 'support' refers to the karma. Sheltering here means that the guna approve of these thoughts,

and say okay to them. Support here means that after we say okay to them, we have the opportunities to fulfill them. Thus, the chitta is said to be the root cause, which leads to the emergence of thoughts. Then these thoughts are liked or disliked. Once they are liked, we accept them as something we want to pursue. Then based on the opportunities we figure out a method by which they can be fulfilled, and then we execute that process of fulfillment. These five stages of progression are called thinking, feeling, willing, knowing, and acting, and they represent how thoughts from the unconscious become conscious activity. After describing this process, this sūtra states that if the unconscious chitta was destroyed, then this process would also terminate.

Sūtra 4.12

अतीतानागतं स्वरूपतोऽस्त्यध्वभेदाद्धर्माणाम्

atītānāgataṁ svarūpato'styadhvabhedāddharmāṇām

atīta—the past; anāgataṁ—the future; svarūpatah—the forms; asti—exist; adhva—uninterrupted; bhedād—their differences; dharmāṇām—their properties or behavior or actions.

TRANSLATION

The past and the future exist uninterrupted as forms (in the present); their differences are known by their properties, behavior, or actions.

COMMENTARY

Our memories exist in the present, but when we recall them, we don't think that what we are experiencing at the moment truly exists at this moment. We somehow know that this experience pertains to the past. Likewise, when we create a vision of the future, we have an experience. But we know that although it is being experienced at present, it pertains to the future. How do we know when some experience at present pertains not to the present, but to the past or the future? The answer is that there are differences in the *form* in how these memories are stored. To understand this idea, we need to distinguish between the *meaning* and the *reference* in a statement. For instance, the statement "the sky is blue" has a meaning, in which 'sky' is a name, and 'blue' is a property. The name 'sky' also has a reference to something outside the sentence. Thus, when we look at the sky, we might have the experience of something bluish. But we don't think that this experience is purely in my head; we think that there is something objective outside my head that is creating this experience. The term 'sky' creates this distinction between my experience and reality; by using this term we indicate that there is something objective outside my observation.

In the same way, our memories also have meaning and reference. The meaning is the recollection of events, and the reference is that it occurred in the past. When we have visions of the future, again, there is an experience, but there is also a reference to something in the future. Our recollections also tell us about the place where something occurred, the individuals who were involved in it, and the situation at that time, etc. In short, the content of our experience carries the references to place, time, individual, and role, and all these are embedded in the same form as the content. These memories are therefore symbols which encode not just the content but also the references to other things as well.

The guna, karma, chitta, etc. comprise such symbols. They are all forms, but the differences in these forms give them their radically different properties.

Sūtra 4.13

ते व्यक्तसूक्ष्मा गुणात्मानः

te vyaktasūkṣmā guṇātmānaḥ

te—they (the past and future); vyaktasūkṣmā—are manifest in the subtle form; guṇātmānaḥ—having the characteristics of the three modes of nature.

TRANSLATION

The past and the future are manifest in the subtle form, having the characteristics of the three modes of nature.

COMMENTARY

The references of the memories or desires can be of the past or the future, but the content of these memories is comprised of the three modes of nature. Even the references—namely, the past, present, and future—are understood as three modes of nature; the past is tamo-guna, the future is rajo-guna, and the present is sattva-guna. Thus, the three modes of nature can be understood both in terms of types that constitute the varieties in space and time. The space variety of guna creates the content, which has spatial references to other things, and the time variety represents the past, present, and future references, along with the types of that time (since each moment in time also has a unique quality).

Sūtra 4.14
परिणामैकत्वाद्वस्तुतत्त्वम्
pariṇāmaikatvādvastutattvam

pariṇāma—the results; ekatvād—oneness; vastu—the real thing; tattvam—essence of.

TRANSLATION
The results have oneness with the essence of the real thing.

COMMENTARY
In any scientific explanation, a distinction is drawn between the phenomena and the reality. The phenomena are those that appear to us, and the reality is that which causes these phenomena. Now, every philosophical system has debated the problem of how to infer the cause from the effects. For example, if you see an apple, does it mean that there is really an apple 'out there' or does it mean that there is something that creates the impression of an apple in us? In modern science, a clear distinction is drawn between phenomena and reality. For example, when you see the redness of an apple, the reality is not red; it is some atoms, and when electrons transition from one state to another, they emit some light which has a particular frequency, which creates the impression of redness. In short, our observations cannot tell us about reality; we have to rather use some theories and models based on inferences to know the nature of reality. If the theory or model is successful in predicting and explaining the observations, then we can tentatively accept the truth of that theory, and the concepts in that theory or model become 'real' for the time being. In short, a distinction between phenomena and reality leads to a permanent distrust in the truth.

Vedic philosophy treats this problem differently; it says that if you are seeing an apple, potentially there is indeed an apple; the exception to that possibility is that you might be hallucinating; however, even if you are hallucinating, there is still something apple-like which causes the impression of an apple. The form of the apple, for instance, exists in your mind, and it can be revived to create the impression of an apple. Therefore, the concept of apple is real, although it may be real in the external world, or merely in the mind. And the cause of experience of the apple is the form of the apple; in this way, the result of observation is identical to the cause, although the cause can be within our minds or outside our minds. In Sāñkhya philosophy, for example, our ordinary perceptual properties like taste, touch, smell, sound, and sight are considered real. Thus, when we taste sweetness, and this is not a hallucination, then the world can objectively be described as the existence of the property of sweetness.

This idea is important because now knowledge is not merely acquired through inference, theory, or model building. Rather, we can directly perceive reality just as it is, because our direct perceptions are not always false.

This sūtra then goes onto state that whatever we experience is caused by something whose essence is identical to what we experience. That essence can be the true nature of how things exist externally or internally. But that essence preexists and causes an experience in us. Thus, even if have a hallucination, the causes of that hallucination have the essence of creating a hallucination. Hence, if we are suffering in life, we can know that there is a cause whose essence is to create suffering. Such essences are comprised of guna and karma. So, the pleasure of eating a fruit can be decomposed into the karma that gives us the fruit, and the guna which gives us the liking for the fruit. The underlying cause of that experience has the essence to create this pleasure, and that pleasure is determined what we like. Thus, our pleasures and pains are not accidental; the effects we see can be traced to an essence which explains its occurrence.

Sūtra 4.15

वस्तुसाम्ये चित्तभेदात्तयोर्वभिक्तःपन्थाः

vastusāmye cittabhedāttayorvibhaktaḥ panthāḥ

vastusāmye—similarity with the real thing; cittabhedāt—due to differences in chitta; tayor—its; vibhaktaḥ—the divisions; panthāḥ—paths.

TRANSLATION

Despite similarity with the real thing (guna and karma), due to differences in the chitta, its divisions create many paths.

COMMENTARY

A good example to illustrate this sūtra is to think of food. Each country has bland and spicy cuisines and different people like to taste them because they are driven by the desire for bland or spicy food. However, the cuisines in each country are also different in taste. Thus, in one sense, people across many countries simply enjoy bland and spicy foods—and it can seem that they are all similar. However, they are also enjoying different flavors within those broad categories. In the same way, the guna give a person the desire to taste spicy or bland food. And within that, there are many varieties of spicy or bland food types. We can classify the food types both by the type of cuisine (e.g., Indian, Chinese, Mexican, Italian, etc.) and flavor (e.g., hot and spicy vs. bland or flavorless). In the same way, we can separate the variety both by the guna and the chitta.

Sūtra 4.16
न चैकचित्ततन्त्रं वस्तु तदप्रमाणकं तदा किं स्यात्
na caikacittatantraṁ vastu tadapramāṇakaṁ tadā kiṁ syāt

na—not; ca—also; eka—one; cittatantraṁ—difference in the chitta; vastu—the real thing; tad—that (result or effect); apramāṇakaṁ—non-proof; tadā—then; kiṁ—what; syāt—happens?

TRANSLATION

One difference in the chitta also doesn't decide that result or effect's non-proof; otherwise, what will happen? (i.e., nothing at all will happen).

COMMENTARY

A child may be attracted to some new toy, although it has no previous experience of that toy, owing to which he has no prior impressions. Just because the prior experience doesn't exist, we cannot preclude the child's attraction to the toy. Conversely, if the child has played a lot with a toy, then it may not be attracted toward the toy, although it has the prior experience of playing with it. Therefore, the non-existence of impressions doesn't preclude the attractions, and the existence of impressions doesn't guarantee them. Sometimes we are drawn toward a thing because of familiarity, and sometimes due to unfamiliarity. This is because the chitta is not the only determinant of experiences. We are also driven by our guna or desires. For instance, if our guna is that of seeking adventure and novelty, then we are naturally drawn toward the unfamiliar. However, if the guna is that of safety and security, then we are drawn toward the unfamiliar. Therefore, one cannot argue that the ultimate result of the experience depends exclusively on the chitta, because guna has a role as well.

Most people unfamiliar with an alien culture, religion, or race tend to avoid the people from that culture, religion, or race, because unfamiliarity makes them scared of the unknown. But sometimes, the unfamiliarity combines with the thrill-seeking tendency, and can make people more eager to know about the alien race, culture, or religion. In this case, the familiarity or the unfamiliarity with some race, culture, or religion is due to the previously formed impressions in the chitta, and the risk-avoiding or thrill-seeking nature is due to the guna. Neither of them alone can determine the outcome. Therefore, singular differences in the chitta do not always determine the outcomes. If that were the case, then the unfamiliar people would never mix, and the familiar people would never separate. The existence of such cases requires both chitta and guna.

Sūtra 4.17

तदुपरागापेक्षत्विाच्चत्तिस्य वस्तु ज्ञाताज्ञातम्

taduparāgāpekṣitvāccittasya vastu jñātājñātam

tad—that; uparāga—conditions; apekṣitvā—the expectation; ca—also; cittasya—of the chitta; vastu—the real thing; jñātājñātam—the familiar and the unfamiliar.

TRANSLATION

That (one difference) also conditions the expectation of the chitta about the familiar and the unfamiliar in the real thing.

COMMENTARY

Even if we mix with an unfamiliar race or culture, we might often seek the comfort of the familiarity. For example, people living in an alien country often visit the places that remind them of their own country. Likewise, even if we live in a familiar race or culture, we often seek the novelty of the unfamiliar. For example, people living in one country like to taste the cuisines of the other nations. Each person has different capacities for novelty and safety, and they become dominant and subordinate at different times. Sometimes novelty drives us toward an experience, and sometimes away from that experience. Likewise, sometimes familiarity drives us toward an experience and sometimes away from it. In this way, the impressions in the chitta 'condition' or 'color' the guna and karma—i.e., they drive us toward something, or push us away from it.

Sūtra 4.18
सदा ज्ञाताश्चित्तवृत्तयस्तत्प्रभोःपुरुषस्यापरिणामित्वात्
sadā jñātāścittavṛttayastatprabhoḥ puruṣasyāpariṇāmitvāt

sadā—always; jñātāh—the familiarity; citta—the chitta; vṛttayastat—the tendencies of that; prabhoḥ—the lord and master; puruṣasya—about the puruṣa; apariṇāmitvāt—as if not having a result.

TRANSLATION
The continuous familiarity with the lord and master, creates the tendencies in the chitta about the Puruṣa, (and those tendencies) do not have a result.

COMMENTARY
The purpose of yoga is not just to cease the thoughts resulting from material impressions, but to form new impressions from which new thoughts can arise. The impressions are about the Supreme Lord. Such impressions do not create karma, and hence this sūtra states that these do not lead to (material) results.

Sūtra 4.19
न तत्स्वाभासं दृश्यत्वात्
na tatsvābhāsaṁ dṛśyatvāt

na—not; tat—that; svābhāsaṁ—the reflection of the self; dṛśyatvāt—due to being seen.

TRANSLATION

Those impressions (formed by the meditation on the Lord) are not seen as being caused by the reflection of the self.

COMMENTARY

The impersonalists contend that meditation on the Lord is merely a route to self-discovery, and by such meditation ultimately one sees oneself as God. This sūtra refutes that contention. The meditation on the Lord reveals the nature of the Lord, and it indirectly reveals the nature of the self as the Lord's devotee. Therefore, it is said that while meditating on the Lord, the self is automatically discovered. That, however, doesn't mean that the self is the object of meditation.

Sūtra 4.20
एकसमये चोभयानवधारणम्
ekasamaye cobhayānavadhāraṇam

ekasamaye—simultaneously; ca—also; ubhaya—the two; anavadhāraṇam—cannot be meditated upon.

TRANSLATION

Also, the two (the soul and the Lord) cannot be simultaneously meditated on.

COMMENTARY

The consciousness of the soul can be either directed toward itself or directed toward the Lord. Even when we perceive a material object, we are not self-aware. We are rather 'lost' in the perception of that specific object. Even in the perception of that object, our consciousness can shift its focus, and alternately focus on sensation, thoughts, judgments, intentions, and values. Similarly, the consciousness can also be withdrawn into the awareness of the self. These types of awareness are mutually exclusive. We can focus on one thing at a time, and thereby, we defocus from the other things. Therefore, the idea that as we meditate on the Lord, we simultaneously become aware of the self is false. The goal of meditation is to direct the consciousness on the Lord, which forms the purpose of life. By living that purpose, we are lost in the experience of the Lord, although through that purpose we enjoy a blissful state of existence. In such a state, the happiness is ours and the soul is lost in the enjoyment of that happiness, which is internal. But the Lord is the object through which that happiness is derived. Therefore, the cognition pertains to the Lord, and the happiness pertains to the self. Apart from these, there is no third experience of 'self' that exists outside of the devotional activities in relationship to the Lord. Therefore, in one sense, the self-identity is forgotten, although that identity is not destroyed.

Sūtra 4.21

चतितान्तरदृश्ये बुद्धबिुद्धेरतिप्रसङ्गःस्मृतसिङ्करश्च

cittāntaradṛśye buddhibuddheratiprasaṅgaḥ smṛtisaṅkaraśca

citta—the chitta; antaradṛśye—in the inner vision; buddhi—the intellect; buddher—the known; atiprasaṅgaḥ—the extreme case; smṛti—memory; saṅkara—being narrow; ca—also.

TRANSLATION

In the inner vision of the chitta, it would be the extreme case of the intellect becoming the known, and also the memory being narrow.

COMMENTARY

The yogi is prescribed withdrawing the consciousness into the self to inculcate detachment from the material world. This situation is not rejected. However, what does one realize by such withdrawing? One comes to know that he is different from the body. This the realization that the soul exists eternally. However, it is not the realization of the life's purpose. Why do we exist? Why should we exist? These questions are not answered by the realization that the self exists eternally. Therefore, the realization of the self is incomplete. The purpose of existence is a deeper-level reality that must also be realized. And that purpose is achieved when the soul is understood as being a part of God. Then three additional kinds of realization are attained— (1) there is a relationship to God, (2) in that relationship there is a mood of love and devotion, and (3) there are activities performed due to that love and devotion. These three kinds of realizations then expand the consciousness away from the self into a spiritual world where there are other devotees of the Lord, who are engaged in various kinds of loving and devotional activities, and as a result they experience various moods of devotional happiness. If the consciousness is restricted to the self, then the broader reality—namely, the whole truth, and the other parts of the whole truth—are not realized. This type of knowledge is restricted or constrained. Therefore, this sūtra doesn't reject the possibility of such withdrawal but considers it to be the 'extreme case' of limiting our self-realization.

Sūtra 4.22
चतिरपरतसिङ्क्रमायास्तदाकारापत्तौ स्वबुद्धिसंवेदनम्
citerapratisaṅkramāyāstadākārāpattau svabuddhisaṁvedanam

citeh—the consciousness; apratisaṅkramāyāh—is toward not being narrowed (i.e., toward expansion); tad—that; ākārāpattau—form is produced; svabuddhi—with own intelligence; saṁvedanam—capacity for emotion.

TRANSLATION
When the consciousness is toward not being narrowed (i.e., toward expansion), that form with its own intelligence and capacity for emotion is produced.

COMMENTARY
The previous sūtra spoke about the extreme case of restricting of the consciousness to the self, and thereby advised its expansion. This sūtra says that when the consciousness is thus expanded, a form of the soul is manifest, which has both cognitive and emotive capacities. The relational capacity was already present as the ability to direct the consciousness to different things. The process of the development of this body is similar to the acquisition of the material body, where the soul's consciousness is distracted toward pradhāna or the idea of greatness, and then the moral sense, ego, intellect, mind, senses, and the body develop as a result of this attraction. Similarly, when the consciousness is attracted toward the Lord, the soul seeks a new kind of greatness—this time the greatness of serving the

Lord perfectly—and based on this quest for greatness, a new type of moral sense, ego, intellect, mind, senses, and the body are developed, which are suited for serving the Lord, in the desired mood and relation. This body or form is called 'sva' or one's own, and not separated from the soul. Hence, the intellect is not material, but svabuddhi or one's own intellect.

Sūtra 4.23
दरष्दृद्दृश्योपरक्तं चत्तिं सर्वार्थम्
drasṭṛdṛśyoparaktaṁ cittaṁ sarvārtham

draṣṭṛ—the seer; dṛśya—the seen; uparaktaṁ—conditioned or influenced by; cittaṁ—the chitta; sarvārtham—all the meanings.

TRANSLATION
(In that state), the seer and the seen are conditioned or influenced by all the meanings in the chitta.

COMMENTARY
As we have discussed before, the chitta represents the concepts of greatness, or ideals, in terms of which we cognize the world, and we try to realize or attain those ideals or greatness in our life. The material notion of greatness is detached from God, and therefore, one seeks to become great like God. One forgets that God is already much greater in all the ways that we are trying to be great and therefore we should serve that greatness. But when the soul directs its consciousness toward the Lord, then it realizes that the true source of greatness is the Lord, because in the Lord all the qualities of greatness are present simultaneously, whereas they were separated in the material nature. Then, the idea of greatness of the self is modified—it is great to serve that greatness.

The ideals of greatness are still present in the chitta, but they are known as the Lord's greatness, rather than as self-greatness. When the moral sense, ego, intellect, mind, the senses, and the body develop from this idea of the Lord's greatness, then everything is imbued with the meaning from which they have sprung. Just like if the cow expands from a mammal, the idea of mammal is present within the cow. Similarly, when the body expands from the meaning of serving the greatness, then every part of the body is imbued with the cognition of the Lord's greatness and the eagerness to please Him. The body is no longer lusting for self-satisfaction; it is rather lusting for the happiness obtained by increasing the Lord's happiness. Such a body never indulges in immoral activities, never produces any karma, is never entangled by the laws of moral action, and hence there is never a need to transmigrate from one body to another.

Sūtra 4.24
तदसङ्ख्येयवासनाभिश्चित्रमपि परार्थं संहत्यकारित्वात्
tadasaṅkhyeyavāsanābhiścitramapi parārtham saṁhatyakāritvāt

tad—that; asaṅkhyeya—innumerable; vāsanābhi—imbued with desires; ca—also; citramapi—even the consciousness; parārtham—the transcendental purpose; saṁhatya—sacrificial; kāritvāt—from the actions.

TRANSLATION
In that state, even the consciousness is imbued with innumerable desires and the actions are performed as sacrifices for the transcendental purpose.

COMMENTARY
The Vedic concept of a sacrifice involves three notions called *soma*, *agni*, and *vāyu*. The soma is our pleasure, the agni is the purpose for which the pleasure is sacrificed, and the vāyu is the process for performing this sacrifice. Thus, the spiritual life is compared to a yajñā in which the soul develops innumerable desires to satisfy the Lord. In this process, whatever the soul finds pleasing, he gives it to the Lord. The judgment of what is good and pleasing is based on the soul's own intelligence; as a result, different souls, who have different kinds of intellects, give different things to the Lord, because they consider them very pleasing. And due to the desire to give these varied things, the desires for giving are also endless. In a material yajñā, one performs a sacrifice to get something in return. But in a spiritual yajñā, one gives out of love, only with the desire to please the Lord, and without the expectation of anything else in return.

Sūtra 4.25

वशिेषदर्शनि आत्मभावभावनावनिवृत्तिः

viśeṣadarśina ātmabhāvabhāvanāvinivṛttiḥ

viśeṣadarśina—seeing the specific distinctions; ātmābhāva—the self-ishness; bhāvanā—the feeling of; vinivṛttiḥ—complete cessation.

TRANSLATION

One who sees the specific distinctions (between material and spiritual sacrifices) attains complete cessation of the feelings of selfishness.

COMMENTARY

The pleasure obtained through a loving sacrifice is incomparable to the pleasure obtained through material sacrifices. First, the results of material sacrifices are governed by karma; therefore, one may work very hard toward a goal and never attain the results. Second, even when the sacrifices are performed, those receiving the results of the sacrifice don't always show gratitude; they feel entitled to receive, but not grateful to receive; this type of sacrifice becomes dissatisfying. Third, the senses are never fully satisfied by such sacrifices because the goal of a material sacrifice is to attain greatness, and sacrifice is contrary to greatness; thus, when some greatness is attained, then one becomes averse to sacrificing, and slowly loses that greatness. The sacrifices for the Lord are different: (a) they are not constrained by karma, (b) the Lord is always grateful and appreciative of the devotees' love, and (c) one is fully satisfied by such performances. Hence, this sūtra states that one who truly understands the differences between material and spiritual sacrifices gives up the attempt to become great through material sacrifices, and devotes himself to the Lord.

Sūtra 4.26

तदा वविेकनम्निनङ्कैवल्यप्राग्भारञ्चतितम्

tadā vivekanimnaṅkaivalyaprāgbhārañcittam

tadā—thereafter; viveka—true knowledge; nimnaṅ—surrendering; kaivalya—liberation; prāgbhārañ—filled with the conclusion; cittam—the chitta.

TRANSLATION

Thereafter, with true knowledge, one surrenders (to the Lord), and the chitta is filled with the conclusion of liberation (from material entanglement).

COMMENTARY

The devotion to the Lord is not whimsical, fanatical, or sentimentality. It is based on a complete understanding of the nature of both material and spiritual realities. Without such knowledge, even if someone fanatically or sentimentally surrenders to the Lord, that surrender is generally temporary. When, instead, the surrender is based on the complete understanding of the nature of the Lord and His various spiritual and material manifestations, then there are no doubts. Instead, the consciousness is imbued with the conviction about the goal of life, and the soul fully dedicates himself toward this purpose. Hence, if one desires to become serious about spiritual attainment, then he must focus on convincing themselves through the acquisition of knowledge of the nature of reality.

Sūtra 4.27

तच्छिद्रेषु प्रत्ययान्तराणि संस्कारेभ्यः
tacchidreṣu pratyayāntarāṇi saṁskārebhyaḥ

tat—in that; chidreṣu—the holes; pratyaya—the qualities, parts, or properties; antarāṇi—within the self; saṁskārebhyaḥ—and the impressions.

TRANSLATION

In those holes (which are left open by the conclusion of liberation), the qualities, parts, or properties, and the impressions appear within the self.

COMMENTARY

Once the final conclusion about the devotion to the Lord is reached, there are still holes in our understanding—these holes pertain to the soul's own role, purpose, and place in the bigger scheme of things. However, if the big picture is known, then the details are filled accurately, and these details are the various qualities, parts, properties, and impressions using which the soul fulfills its purpose of existence. In the material world also, the soul begins with the conclusion—e.g., that

I am great—and the details pertain to how one becomes great. These details manifest after the conclusion is reached. Hence, the material body appears as a consequence of the soul's attempt at greatness. Similarly, when the soul reaches the conclusion that the Lord is the greatest, and the soul's purpose is to serve the Lord, then details appear. These details pertain to how the soul must serve the Lord, through which relationship, and with which qualities.

Sūtra 4.28
हानमेषां क्लेशवदुक्तम्
hānameṣāṁ kleśavaduktam

hānameṣāṁ—in this way are destroyed; kleśavat—all that is just like painful; uktam—it is stated.

TRANSLATION
All the painful experiences are destroyed in this way; thus, it is said.

COMMENTARY
The greatest crisis in our lives is the ignorance of who we are, why we are here, what is the purpose of our lives, and how to attain perfect happiness. This crisis cannot be resolved by mundane means. We can accumulate any amount of wealth, followers, name and fame, power, relatives, and friends, and we can use these avenues as distractions to forget about the crisis in our lives. But this crisis always returns, because the distractions that make us forget about the crisis are always temporary. The permanent solution to this crisis is that we revive our relationship to the Lord. Then, whether we are in this world or another world, in this body or another body, there is perfect clarity about who we are, why we are here, the purpose of our lives, and how to become perfectly happy. Once this crisis is resolved, then gradually all other painful things are destroyed. The clarity of purpose in life mitigates the pain out of most sufferings, and whatever small suffering remains also disappears gradually over time.

Sūtra 4.29
प्रसङ्ख्यानेऽप्यकुसीदस्य सर्वथा विविकख्यातेर्धर्ममेघःसमाधिः
**prasaṅkhyāne'pyakusīdasya sarvathā
vivekakhyāterdharmameghaḥ samādhiḥ**

prasaṅkhyāne—in the perfect knowledge of Sāṅkhya; api—even;
akusīdasya—this thing without any gain; sarvathā—completely; viveka—
true knowledge; khyāter—that is renowned; dharmameghaḥ—the cloud
of dharma; samādhiḥ—perfectly absorbed in meditation and the same as
the origin.

TRANSLATION
Even in the perfect knowledge of Sāṅkhya, this thing without any
gain is completely (destroyed). With true knowledge that is renowned as
the cloud of dharma (i.e., it quenches the fire of material existence), one
becomes fully absorbed in perfect meditation and becomes the same as
the origin.

COMMENTARY
This sūtra refers to the virtues of the Sāṅkhya philosophy, which provides the knowledge to discriminate between material and spiritual, the
various pathways for elevating the soul from the present condition, the
nature of the perfectional state, and how the soul lives in a different kind
of spiritual body. The conclusions of these two philosophies are identical
(indeed, the conclusions of all Vedic systems of philosophies are identical).
There are minor differences in the details about how one must practice
regulations to attain this perfection.

Sūtra 4.30
ततःक्लेशकर्मनिवृत्तिः
tataḥ kleśakarmanivṛttiḥ

tataḥ—from that (knowledge of Sāṅkhya); kleśa—the suffering;
karma—of karma; nivṛttiḥ—cessation of.

TRANSLATION
From the knowledge of Sāṅkhya, the suffering of karma ceases.

COMMENTARY

The Yoga Sūtras have described an eight-fold process beginning with Yama and Niyama to finally absorption in the meditation of the Lord. The Sāñkhya Sūtras prescribe other methods such as the chanting of mantras, leading a regulated life of Varṇāśrama, etc. ultimately culminating in devotion to the Lord. Therefore, the initial steps in these systems are clearly different, but the final conclusion about the goal of life, or what must be attained by these practices, is the same. In this way, there are many systems of religiosity prescribed in the Vedic texts, and this diversity tends to confuse people—only if they don't understand that these are different paths to the same destination. The Vedic system is very definitive about the goal, but prescribes many optional paths to attain this goal. These paths are also not the only possible paths. One can also combine these paths, use them alternately, or even follow other paths—under the guidance of an enlightened spiritual master. Such a spiritual master knows how to adapt and adjust the various paths to the needs of a specific individual. As long as the ultimate goal is attained, all the paths are considered good.

Sūtra 4.31

तदा सर्वावरणमलापेतस्य ज्ञानस्यानन्त्याज्ज्ञेयमल्पम्

tadā sarvāvaraṇamalāpetasya jñānasyānantyājjñeyamalpam

tadā—then; sarva—all; āvaraṇa—coverings; mala—of impurities; apetasya—are removed; jñāna—by knowledge; asya—of that; anantyāt—from the infinite; jñeyam—is known; alpam—the small things.

TRANSLATION

Then, all coverings of impurities are removed by knowledge from that infinite; by knowing (that infinite) all the small things (are known).

COMMENTARY

The materialist-reductionist believes that the knowledge of the overall purpose of life would be decided by the study of atoms and molecules. However, this sūtra inverts that process and states that once the big picture is known, then then the details are automatically understood. Therefore, the Vedic system is not opposed to the study of material details such as atoms, space, time, causality, etc. But all these studies are done within the context of the overall conclusion that the soul is different from the body, that its purpose is devotion to the Lord, and it is entangled in this world due to the forgetfulness of this purpose. This forgetfulness creates many kinds of perceptual and conceptual 'impurities' which narrowly focus the consciousness into the details, all the while keeping the soul forgetful about the big purpose of life. One symptom of this impurity is that people spend most of their lives worrying about the well-being of their, family, children, job, parents, wealth, and comfortable accommodation, and the pleasures that life can afford them, and deprioritize the spiritual pursuits. They think that once all these minor details are worked out, then they will focus on the big picture of life. But the reality is that such an outcome never transpires. All the time is lost in mundane activities, the attachment to these things grows, and one is unable to control the mind and the senses. At the point of death, all these impressions created during this life cause rebirth into another life. If the dominant impressions in this life are materialistic, then the next life simply perpetuates that materialism. Therefore, all Vedic scriptures advise that one should fix the big picture first, and worry about the minor details subsequently.

Sūtra 4.32
तत:कृतार्थानां परिणामक्रमसमाप्तिर्गुणानाम्
tataḥ kṛtārthānāṁ pariṇāmakramasamāptirguṇānām

tataḥ—thereafter; kṛtārthānāṁ—having accomplished the purpose; pariṇāma—the results; krama—sequential; samāptir—the end of; guṇānām—the material modes of nature.

TRANSLATION
Thereafter, having accomplished the purpose (of purification), the sequential results of the material modes of nature come to an end.

COMMENTARY
The process of yoga described earlier described a sequence of events in which the chitta is purified of the modes of nature, then the soul comes to know about the Lord, and finally, by this knowledge, the karma is

destroyed. The process of Sāṅkhya described here changes that sequence somewhat. It states that by engaging in devotional activities, one's karma is completely destroyed, then one obtains an understanding of the Lord, and finally, all the guna are destroyed. In this way, Yoga and Sāñkhya are complementary systems. In the former, guna is destroyed before karma, and in the latter, karma is destroyed before guna. The ultimate destruction of guna and karma is mediated by the perfect knowledge of the Lord. Therefore, one can practice either of these methods, or both methods in combination. They produce the same outcomes.

Sūtra 4.33

कषणपरतयोगी परणिामापरान्तनरि्गर्राह्यःक्रमः

kṣaṇapratiyogī pariṇāmāparāntanirgrāhyaḥ kramaḥ

kṣaṇa—moments in time; pratiyogī—by the cooperation of; pariṇāma—the results; aparānta—the termination of the inferior; nirgrāhyaḥ—a state that cannot be perceived; kramaḥ—the sequence.

TRANSLATION

The results are produced by the cooperation of the moments in time; upon the termination of the inferior, the sequence (in time) becomes unperceivable.

COMMENTARY

The spiritual world is called parā, and the material world is called aparā. In this aparā world, time is the primary cause of effects. For example, time manifests the desires from guna, the impressions from the chitta, and the opportunities from the karma. The soul simply has the choice to reject these automatically created effects. Therefore, the soul is bound by the action of time, and the laws of nature. In the parā world, this effect of time doesn't exist. Rather, the desires, impressions, and opportunities are created simply by the soul's desires. Therefore, in a simple sense, the liberation from material existence means the liberation from the effect of time. Once the soul is freed from guna and karma, and the chitta has been purified, the sequence of the moments in time has no effect. This is the ultimate cessation of all forms of material causation and the freedom from the laws of nature. Time is now the succession of the soul's choices, and it can go slower or faster, or even stop completely, based on the soul's choices. Thus, whatever is enjoyable is incessantly elongated by the soul's desires, and whatever is not enjoyable is never chosen, because that time never arrives.

Sūtra 4.34

पुरुषार्थशून्यानां गुणानां प्रतिप्रसवःकैवल्यं स्वरूपप्रतिष्ठा वा चितिशक्तिरिति

puruṣārthaśūnyānāṁ guṇānāṁ pratiprasavaḥ kaivalyaṁ svarūpapratiṣṭhā vā citiśaktiriti

puruṣārtha—the purpose of mankind; śūnyānāṁ—nothingness; guṇānāṁ—of the modes of nature; pratiprasavaḥ—toward their stage of birth; kaivalyaṁ—the liberation; svarūpapratiṣṭhā—being situated in one's true form; vā—moved; citiśaktir—by the power of consciousness; iti—in conclusion.

TRANSLATION

In conclusion, the purpose of mankind is the taking the modes of nature toward their stage of birth from nothingness, and liberation is being situated in one's true form, moving by the power of consciousness.

COMMENTARY

The entire Yoga Sūtra is summarized in this conclusion. The variety of the material body arises from a deep-seated, but false, notion of greatness. This idea of greatness is called pradhāna, or that "I am God", and there is nothing other than me. It is a state of voidness, because nothing else is known—there is ignorance about the nature of the Lord, and unawareness of other living entities. In short, the self is personalized, matter is depersonalized, and God and other souls are voided. Under this false idea that "only I exist, and everything is meant for me" the material world is manifest. The purpose of the process of yoga is to reverse the process of creation and take it to that point of origin, where the soul's false egotism is manifest. Then, this false egotism must be uprooted, and the true ego of the soul—as the servant of the Lord—can be established. The liberated state is not formless, or devoid of other individuals. Rather, if we understand the cause of material creation, then the depersonalization of nature, and the voiding of other individuals (including God) is part of the materialistic ego. Thus, those who try to attain such impersonalistic or voidistic realities remain within the material condition, whereas those who try to uproot the main cause of the material entanglement become liberated from matter.

Index